Eat Your Heart Out

Eat Your Heart Out

The Fallacy of the Healthy Diet

Dr James Le Fanu

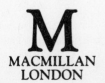

MACMILLAN
LONDON

To Juliet

First published 1987 by
MACMILLAN LONDON LIMITED
4 Little Essex Street London WC2R 3LF
and Basingstoke

Associated companies in Auckland, Delhi, Dublin, Gaborone, Hamburg, Harare, Hong Kong, Johannesburg, Kuala Lumpur, Lagos, Manzini, Melbourne, Mexico City, Nairobi, New York, Singapore and Tokyo

British Library Cataloguing in Publication Data
Le Fanu, James
  Eat your heart out: the fallacy of the healthy diet.
  1. Nutrition
  I. Title
  613.2   TX353

  ISBN 0-333-44202-4

Typeset by Rowland Phototypesetting Limited
Bury St Edmunds, Suffolk

Printed by Anchor Brendon Limited, Tiptree, Essex

Contents

Foreword

Medicine being the compendium of the successive and contradictory mistakes of medical practitioners, when we summon the wisest of them to our aid, the chances are we may be relying on a scientific truth, the error of which will be recognised in a few years' time.
(Marcel Proust: *À la recherche du temps perdu*)

This book refutes the conventional wisdom that the food we eat is an important cause of disease and death in our society – the diet-disease thesis. It does so by showing that the scientific evidence employed by its protagonists to sustain their arguments does not stand up to critical scrutiny.

It does not argue that the foods currently claimed to be harmful are in fact beneficial, or indeed the reverse. Rather it demonstrates that, as far as present knowledge allows, food is simply not an important or modifiable cause of disease in our society.

So although the focus is on nutrition, the interest lies in the misuse of science. Not the misuse that has scientists undertaking sinister experiments or fabricating their results, but the misuse whereby false theories are constructed out of a partial or less than fully straightforward interpretation of facts.

There is a further interest. In investigating one section of the diet-disease thesis, the diet-heart thesis that would have heart disease caused by too much fat, that is meat and dairy foods, it became apparent that there is sufficient evidence to suggest a better unifying biological explanation for the disease that has not apparently been noted before. So besides criticising prevailing theories, it is possible at least tentatively to proffer an alternative.

Obviously individual scientists will feature in this account. The protagonists of the thesis come in for considerable criticism, but they are quite able to defend themselves. I have freely quoted from the opinions and statements of those who have been critical of the thesis, but would not want to suggest in any way that they necessarily endorse the wider ideas expressed.

1
Reasons for Doubt

*Western food is the chief cause of the modern epidemic of heart
disease.* (Professor Geoffrey Rose)

*The greatest of all follies is to believe passionately the palpably not
true.* (H. L. Mencken)

The connection between food and disease has always been a happy
hunting ground for quackery. Food's strong psychological, cultural
and sexual connotations, its ubiquity and variety make it a fertile
source of 'explanations' of illness. Over the last 100 years each of its
main constituents, carbohydrate, protein and fat, has at different
times been both incriminated as harmful and promoted as uniquely
beneficial. As long as people are neurotic and unhappy, food quacks
will find a constituency, while the rest of the world can wisely and
safely ignore their admonitions.

But over the last ten years the incrimination of food as an
important cause of illness has received the stamp of approval from
the orthodox medical establishment, and radical changes in the
nation's diet have been encouraged with just as much zeal as by less
orthodox predecessors. Dozens of expert committees have examined the entrails of the scientific evidence and declared unani-
mously that, were we to eat less meat and dairy produce, and more
vegetables and cereals, we would be less prone to suffer a wide
range of illnesses. In particular, the advice goes, we would reduce
our risk of succumbing to heart disease or cancer. In a more popular

version, these dietary recommendations proscribe 'junk' foods – hamburgers, chips and meat pies – as being specifically lethal.

The public is rightly sceptical of the motives and admonitions of experts – but the authority and consistency with which this thesis has been promoted cannot help but have influenced the perceptions of those who would not normally be impressed. Even the most cynical might now be excused feelings of anxiety and guilt when eating many of the foods previously highly esteemed in our culture for their subtlety and sensuousness – the Sunday joint, cream teas and exotic cheeses.

The successful promotion of the diet-disease thesis has extended the influence of medicine well beyond the traditional confines of the GP's surgery and the hospital ward, to reach out and affect the lives of all ordinary citizens, encouraging and cajoling them into making major changes in their lives. The contents of this book will provide succour to those who resent such intrusions.

The main distinguishing feature between the food faddists of the past and the edicts of contemporary expert committees is that the latter are at least well furnished with facts – a veritable cornucopia of them. Over the last thirty years scientists and investigators have been out in the field weighing the stools of the Bantu, measuring the height of the Japanese, taking blood for cholesterol estimations from everybody and finding out what people die from. But facts are tricky things. In abundance they can be used to obscure and mystify and, just as a journalist can select his sources and edit his material to produce a misleading article, so scientists can select and edit facts to substantiate a misleading thesis. Their credibility is enhanced by our scientific culture, in which the suggestions of scientists carry more authority than the opinions of even the most informed and intelligent of the non-scientific laity. Against such a background, why should the public suspect it is being misled; and how can it defend itself?

Common sense is a useful ally. In contemporary Britain most people live out their natural lifespan of a little over threescore years and ten, while at the same time everybody has to die of something. Four out of five deaths from heart disease and cancer occur in people over the age of sixty-five and include many dying quietly of 'old age' in their beds; so when experts claim there is an 'epidemic' of 'diet-related killer diseases', they are likely to be exaggerating. Or again common sense reminds us that we live in a world made up of different races and peoples who are born, grow up, work, and have their own children sustained by a bewildering array of dietary habits. Humans are uniquely capable of this type of biological adaptation and it is therefore most unlikely either that there is something specifically lethal about the Western diet (associated as it is with maximum longevity) or that there might be such a thing as an 'ideal diet' which would somehow confer near-immortality on all who adopted it.

An understanding of the limits of medical knowledge is also helpful. The biology of humans and their diseases is of a fearsome complexity; indeed, outside the infectious and genetic diseases, it is possible to identify a specific cause for less than one per cent of the illnesses in the medical textbook. Medicine's strength has been not in understanding 'causes', but in the empirical treatment of diseases. It is possible to treat diabetes with insulin without knowing what causes it, just as it is possible to drive a car without knowing the principles which govern the internal combustion engine. This is true across the whole spectrum of medicine – so when experts claim that not one but many complex diseases are caused by the food we eat and can be prevented by changing to a 'healthier' diet, they are likely to be misleading the public.

A grasp of history offers a further bulwark against the thesis. Fifty years ago the public was being advised by the experts of the day to increase dramatically its consumption of dairy foods; today it is being advised to reduce them drastically. This change of heart is at least as likely to be explicable in terms of scientific 'fashion' as to be based on hard scientific knowledge. After all, much scientific consensus in the past has subsequently been shown to be in error. At the turn of the century, for instance, in the period immediately following the discovery of bacteria as an important cause of disease but before the discovery of vitamins, numerous illnesses subsequently found to be due to vitamin deficiency were attributed to 'chronic bacterial infection' and treated accordingly. The major site of 'chronic infection' in the body was thought to be the teeth, and so the standard treatment for many diseases became dental extraction. Such was the case with pernicious anaemia, a chronic and debilitating illness due to the failure to absorb the vitamin B_{12}. Before the empirical discovery in the 1930s that the disease was curable by giving its victims large quantities of B_{12}-rich liver, many were rendered toothless – which did nothing to halt the progress of their disease, but certainly added to the distress of their last few years. It is conceivable, therefore, that diet-disease advice may be not only ineffective but also harmful.

Dissension is another guide to weaknesses in the prevailing

orthodoxy. There is much disagreement in medicine, but rarely over well-substantiated practices. Nobody will contest that an inflamed appendix has to be removed urgently, or that a life-threatening pneumonia requires powerful antibiotics. There are, however, many distinguished scientists and doctors who dispute those expert committees which say there is overwhelming evidence that reducing consumption of certain foods will save 'tens of thousands of lives each year'. The arguments of these doubters merit serious attention.

Finally, it is necessary to appreciate that doctors and scientists have to earn a living. Although they may conceal it under a guise of disinterested professionalism and white-coated compassion, they are ultimately governed by the same exigencies as the car salesman – the need to sell their goods in the market place. A degree of scepticism about the motives of the medical profession is only sensible when countering its claims to wisdom.

Common sense, historical understanding, scepticism may do something to thwart the ambitions of experts who wish to change our lives for our own benefit, but at the back of most people's minds there will remain a suspicion that there must be *something*, some substance, to the claims of the diet-disease protagonists. However much common sense may contradict their claims, no one wants to be the smartest corpse in the graveyard. In refuting them, therefore, it is necessary to grapple with the arguments as they are put forward, with the scientific facts, the scientific method and the graphs and tables of scientific presentation.

The central pillar of the diet-disease thesis is the diet-heart hypothesis: that too much fat in the diet, in the form of meat and dairy foods, clogs up the arteries to the heart, leading to a heart attack. This belief is held to be so obvious that it might appear merely perverse to challenge it. Nonetheless it arises from certain scientific observations, so it is only appropriate to examine the basis of those observations. Two pieces of evidence are frequently cited in support of the hypothesis. The first is that Japanese immigrants to the United States change their diet and so acquire the American pattern of heart disease. The second is that the decline in heart disease in the US over the last two decades is due to 'healthier eating'.

The Japanese migrants to the US have been an endless source of fascination for those investigating the causes of disease because as they move they lose the pattern of disease of their native land and acquire that of their adopted country. Thus, while heart disease is rare among Japanese in Japan it is common among Japanese in the US, which is strongly suggestive of some environmental cause for the disease. One obvious possibility is that in the course of moving the migrants have changed their dietary habits to those of their new culture and so increased their susceptibility to certain kinds of illnesses. The main distinguishing feature between the diets of the two countries is that the Japanese eat little fat in the form of meat and dairy produce and so get around 12 per cent of their calories from this source, while in the US these foods are consumed in abundance and provide about 40 per cent of calorie intake.

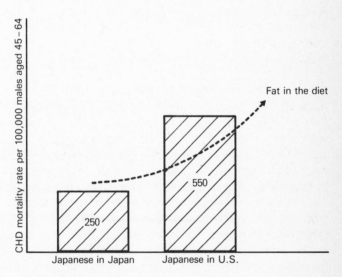

Fig.1.1 *The rate of heart disease increases in Japanese migrants to the United States as they increase the amount of fat in their diet*

The consequences are clearly demonstrated in Fig. 1.1.[1] The hatched columns contrast the rates of heart disease among Japanese in Japan with those of Japanese in the US, while the change in their dietary pattern is shown by an arrow.

So far, so good. But the Japanese have not been the only migrants to the US in the last fifty years: what, then, has been the experience of migrants from other countries? Sweden, for instance, has a similar dietary pattern to America but half the rate of heart disease. Yet when Swedes move to the US they also acquire the US pattern

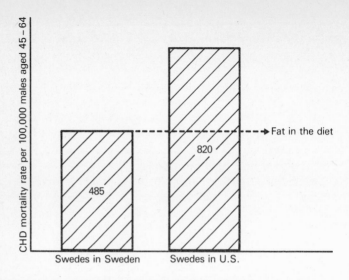

Fig.1.2 *The rate of heart disease rises in Swedish migrants to the United States, even though the amount of fat in their diet remains the same*

of heart disease – that is, the rate markedly increases even though their dietary pattern changes little. This is shown in Fig. 1.2.[2]

Thus, although the experience of the Japanese is often presented as specific evidence of a relation between diet and heart disease, it is in fact only a reflection of a generalised (and for the moment unexplained) phenomenon, that migrants from any country will tend to acquire the pattern of disease of their adopted country. More importantly, the Swedish experience appears actually to *refute* the specific argument that fat intake causes heart disease, because if this were the case then the rate of heart disease among Swedish migrants should have remained the same as that of their country of origin and not markedly increased to match the rates present in the US.

If the evidence from migrant studies is contradictory, what about one of the other main planks of the diet-heart hypothesis – the decline in incidence in heart disease in the US over the last fifteen years? This well-publicised phenomenon has been noted to have occurred dramatically and uniformly across all classes of US society, and is shown in Fig. 1.3.[3] From 1968 to 1984 the mortality rate from the disease among males has fallen by over one-third. This startling pattern has been widely attributed to changes in US 'lifestyle' and

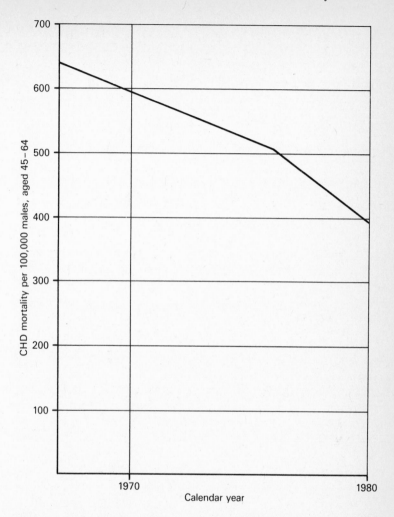

Fig.1.3 *There has been a marked decline in heart disease (CHD) in the United States since 1968*

particularly to changes to a healthier diet. However, examination of the decline of heart disease not only in the US but in several other countries since 1950 offers a more interesting picture. Fig. 1.4 shows that in these countries, almost simultaneously, the rate of heart disease suddenly stopped rising in the mid-1960s and started to fall precipitately and dramatically. Are we expected to believe that in

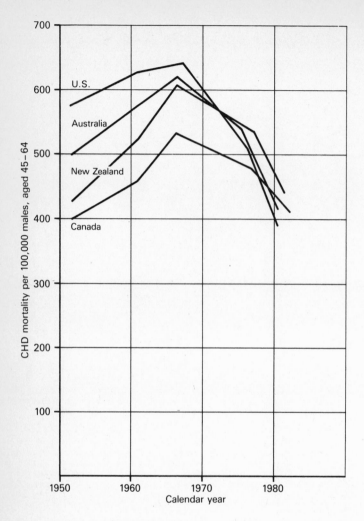

Fig.1.4 *There is a striking similarity in the pattern of heart disease in the U.S., Australia, Canada and New Zealand from 1950 to 1985*

all these countries simultaneously people radically changed their diet and so influenced the subsequent pattern of the disease?

What has really happened to their consumption of dairy foods? As Fig. 1.5 reveals over the period of these changes in heart disease there has in fact been very little change in dietary patterns in these countries.[4] So as with the example of the Swedish migrants, not only

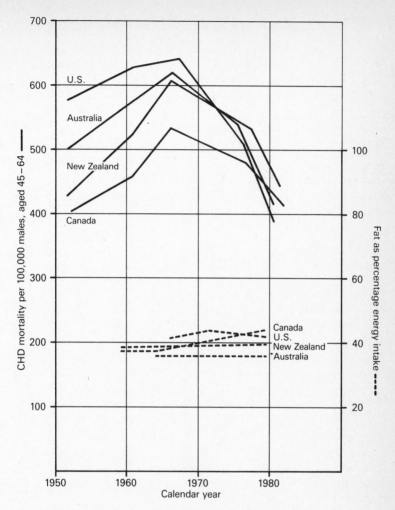

Fig.1.5 *The rise and fall of heart disease has occurred with little change in the amount of fat in the diet*

does a more detailed examination of the evidence fail to confirm the original inference, but it actually appears to refute the notion which in its original form it was being used to prove: that heart disease is related to diet.

In a few paragraphs, then, the diet-heart hypothesis is in deep trouble. This is not because anything its protagonists say is factually incorrect; not at all. It is just that their selection of the evidence is overwhelmingly partial, and the inference drawn from that evidence is unwarranted. The example of the Japanese migrants is much quoted, and the conclusions drawn from it widely propagated; but the same evidence for the Swedes, which contradicts those conclusions, is only to be found by delving back sixteen years into the scientific literature. Similarly, it is not incorrect that the rate of heart disease has been falling in the US, but it is necessary to get out the calculator and the international statistics to find that a similar phenomenon has occurred in several other countries simultaneously, and then to go elsewhere again with the calculator to find that the food consumption statistics which show that the changing pattern of heart disease is not in fact reflected in major changes in diet.

'Lies, damned lies and statistics'? These examples raise the very important issue of whether any conclusions based on the manipulation of statistical data can ever be trusted. Luckily there is an answer to this problem. It is as possible as it is necessary to distinguish between selectively assembled scientific facts and scientific certainties, and a reliable method of doing so was established in the early days of the discovery that bacteria were an important cause of disease.

In 1882 Robert Koch identified the tubercle bacillus as the cause of tuberculosis, and over the next few years, with the simple techniques of staining biological tissues and looking down a microscope, most of the bacteria that cause human disease were discovered. The 'germ theory' of disease was in the ascendant and the centuries-long belief that had attributed illness to the 'miasma' or the 'humours' was swept away.

Very soon a specific germ or bacterium was being sought as the cause of each and every illness, and amidst all the enthusiasm error was inevitable: staining techniques can be faulty, smudges down the microscope can be deceptive and the human mind has a powerful influence over what the eye perceives. In particular, 'bacteria' were alleged to cause many diseases that we now know to be due to vitamin deficiency.

The possibility of error raised the fundamental question of how a scientist could be certain that what he was seeing down the microscope really was the cause of the disease under investigation. It was a question that had already been answered by Koch himself in what have subsequently become known as 'Koch's postulates'. They can be summarised as follows:

1. It is necessary to show that the bacterium considered to cause the disease is present in all cases of the disease.

2. The bacterium must be shown to be a living organism and distinguishable from all other micro-organisms.

3. The bacterium must be capable of being grown outside the diseased person in a specialised medium.

4. The bacterium must, when inoculated into test animals, display the same or similar symptoms to those that it produces in humans.[5]

This last stipulation is especially important as it involves the distinguishing feature of science – the ability to test beliefs by submitting them to the rigour of experiment. If bacterium *a* really is the cause of disease *a*, then the only certain way of demonstrating this is to inject the organism into a test animal and look for evidence of the disease. An experiment is the necessary and logical development of theory, and requires manipulating the external world in a way that will produce definitive, measurable evidence that the theory is correct.

The results of the scientific experiment are the gold standard or 'bottom line' of the scientific enterprise. No matter how much one believes a theory to be true, if it fails the rigours of the experiment, the basis of the beliefs that inspired it must be re-examined and other avenues explored.

To some extent, of course, Koch's postulates are only common sense. If a bacterium isolated from an individual with a disease really is the cause of that disease, then it must fulfil his criteria. If it does not, it is coincidental to the disease process, and other explanations must be sought for the disease under investigation.

When we turn to the evidence for a causal relationship between diet and disease, we find an analogous set of rules which are even more important than Koch's postulates, because the kind of evidence available is even more vulnerable to error than the vogue for discovering non-existent bacteria as the cause of vitamin-deficiency diseases. Here the problem is not one of misconstruing what is seen down the microscope, but of misinterpreting statistical data.

The major source of evidence for the diet-disease thesis comes from a branch of medicine known as Epidemiology, which attempts to relate specific diseases to possible environmental causes. Take a disease, measure its incidence, find out who dies from it, and then look at the lives of its victims and see if there is something that distinguishes them from other people who do not succumb to the disease. In this process certain 'risk factors' for a disease will be identified – that is, certain aspects in the lives of those with the disease, not present in those without it, which might explain why they have contracted it. For example, most cases of lung cancer are found in those with the risk factor of having smoked heavily for many years. Centrally, however, these risk factors are not necessarily the *cause* of the disease; they could merely be *associated* with it.

The distinction is crucial. Imagine, for example, that an investigating epidemiologist, ignorant of Koch's discoveries, were to have gone to Ireland at the end of the last century in search of the cause of tuberculosis. He finds that the disease is commonest among the poorest classes, who also eat a lot of potatoes. He might then suggest that eating potatoes causes the disease, with this series of arguments:

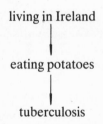

But he would of course only be demonstrating an *association* – namely that poverty, deprivation and overcrowding are associated both with dependence on a cheap home-grown crop, potatoes, and with tuberculosis:

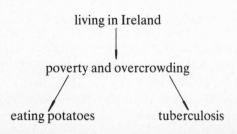

Alternatively, a risk factor might identify an additional but not determinant cause of a disease. Smoking is, for example, a risk factor for death from Legionnaire's disease – a type of pneumonia caused by a bacterium – which has fatal consequences predominantly among those whose lungs are additionally damaged by the ravages of tobacco smoke.

The distinction between 'association' and 'causality' is obviously of fundamental importance, and the tendency to confuse them is the source of all those theories which have at different times implicated so many diseases with each and every aspect of our lives: having cats or central heating, drinking coffee or alcohol, eating gherkins or cauliflowers. Fortunately, however, the dangers of failing to make the all-important distinction, and thereby of developing false theories of the nature of disease, were recognised by the founding father of the discipline of epidemiology, Sir Austin Bradford Hill. In the early 1950s he drew up a series of 'canons', analogous to Koch's postulates, which had to be fulfilled in order to determine whether the relationship between an environmental phenomenon and a disease was genuinely causal or merely associative.[6]

We can see how the method works with the example of smoking and lung cancer. Epidemiological evidence shows that lung cancer predominantly affects smokers. Thus, smoking is a risk factor for the disease; but how can we be sure that they contract the disease because they smoke, and not merely that people who smoke also get lung cancer? The answer is that the evidence to relate smoking and lung cancer fulfils Bradford Hill's canons.[7]

1. *The correlation is biologically plausible:* there are cancer-inducing agents in tobacco that, when brought in contact with lung tissue, could cause the disease.
2. *The correlation is strong:* the death rate from lung cancer in cigarette smokers is ten times higher than in non-smokers.
3. *The correlation reflects a biological gradient:* the more cigarettes that are smoked, the higher the risk of lung cancer.
4. *The correlation is found consistently:* thirty-six separate studies examining the relationship between smoking and lung cancer have found a positive correlation.
5. *The correlation holds over time:* as cigarette consumption has steadily increased it has been paralleled by a rise in incidence of the disease.

6. *The association is confirmed by experiment:* according to Bradford Hill, 'Here the strongest support for a causative hypothesis will be found.' As smoking causes lung cancer, stopping smoking reduces that risk; and the longer the time elapses since stopping smoking, the lower is that risk.

So we have moved from a scientific fact – that people who smoke get lung cancer – to a scientific certainty – that smoking causes lung cancer. Bradford Hill's canons would only have been fulfilled were that the case. There might of course be additional causes for the disease. A rare type of lung cancer can occur in non-smokers. The disease is commoner in urban than rural areas, so perhaps pollution plays a role. Not everyone who smokes gets the disease; perhaps certain people are protected in some way by their genes. But these observations are insufficient to annul the massive, overpowering statistical evidence that smoking causes the disease. By comparison, the association between potato consumption and tuberculosis would not begin to fulfil the criteria; it is not biologically plausible, there is no biological gradient and so on.

As with smoking and lung cancer, the evidence in favour of the diet-heart hypothesis rests on statistics; likewise, it can be tested by Bradford Hill's canons. If the thesis is correct, it should be possible to show that those who get heart disease eat more meat and dairy products than those who do not, and that the more animal fats consumed, the greater the risk of the disease. There should be a correlation over time, so that the increase in heart disease in the Western world this century should be reflected in increasing dairy food and meat consumption; and its decline, in the US and elsewhere, should be reflected in decreasing consumption of these foods. And, crucially, the thesis should be testable by experiment: encouraging people to reduce their fat consumption should demonstrably reduce their subsequent risk of the disease.

If one wanted to simplify the issue it is enough to go to the bottom line, to the last of the canons – the experiment – and inquire of those who advocate a change of diet as a means of preventing heart disease: 'That's all very well but if I do stop eating one lot of food and start eating another, what experiments are there that will show I will actually benefit?'

And now it is possible to see how selection of facts can lead to error. If the protagonists of the diet-heart thesis cite the experience of the Japanese migrants to the US, but omit to mention the results of the Swedish migrants, likewise omitting to point out that the hypothesis does not fulfil Hill's canons and in particular fails the test of experiment, then they are seriously misleading the public.

As will be seen in the relevant chapters, not only does the evidence in favour of the diet-heart thesis fail to show what its protagonists claim for it but, crucially, the thesis does not begin to fulfil Hill's canons. It is through demonstrating this that one is able to refute the thesis. This should be of some interest.

Yet the ability to refute the thesis necessarily raises other questions. Why have the protagonists selected the evidence in a partial way and ignored what contradicts it? How has the deception been orchestrated? Why has it proved so popular? What are the problems in contemporary medicine that have allowed its wide acceptance?

These questions require specific answers, but can also usefully be seen as reflecting recurrent problems of the misuse of science. Conveniently for the argument, the expert committees of fifty years ago were making recommendations that are the exact reverse of current contemporary wisdom, emphasising the need for the nation not to decrease consumption of meat and dairy foods but markedly to increase their consumption. As will be seen, there is a striking resemblance between the methods of argument, the selection of facts, the replacement of reason with rhetoric used by our contemporary experts and those of the 1930s, even though the conclusions they come to are so diverse.

The story starts in the recent past when a group of experts convened to produce a report encouraging the public to change their diet, and the difficulty they had in coping with the rather embarrassing fact that when these recommendations had been critically tested in a series of massive experiments, they had been found not to work.

2
Fat is Harmful – Official

In the summer of 1982 the World Health Organization published a report calling for fundamental changes in the Western diet.[1] It had convened its experts to review the evidence that had been accumulated over the previous twenty years to link heart disease – the commonest cause of early death in males in the Western world – with the consumption of 'saturated fat' (essentially meat and dairy foods). The experts found the evidence convincing, and concluded that in order to prevent the disease, the consumption of the incriminated foods would have to fall by one-third. This meant rationing meat to a few meals per week, replacing whole milk with skimmed, avoiding 'high-fat' cheeses like Cheddar and Camembert, abjuring butter and treating with caution many of the foods highly esteemed in our culture, from salami to pastries.

Four months later, in October, the results were released of an experiment that had been set up to see whether such dietary restrictions would indeed prevent heart disease. Under the headline 'Heart Attacks: A Test Collapses', the *Wall Street Journal* announced: 'After ten years and 115 million dollars one of the largest medical experiments ever attempted has come to nought.'[2]

The experiment, known by the acronym of 'MRFIT' (Multiple Risk Factor Intervention Trial), had been set up in the US to provide proof that dietary changes would reduce the risk of heart attack; but that proof had not been forthcoming. Despite enormous efforts in encouraging 6,000 men for almost a decade to change their diets and stop smoking, the human guinea pigs had exactly the same rate of heart disease as a similar number of men in a control group which had not been so encouraged.[3]

Six months later, at the beginning of 1983, a similar experiment, but this time involving 40,000 men from five different European countries, produced the same verdict: the encouragement of changes in diet did not prevent or reduce the incidence of heart disease.[4]

The behaviour of the WHO expert committee in the summer of 1982 would thus appear to require some explanation. Its members would certainly have known the results of these experiments in advance of publication because they had been actively involved in setting them up. But rather than waiting for publication, the committee anticipated the results by asserting with authority the opposite of what the experiments were actually about to reveal.

Perhaps they thought the results were not important, or that the trials had in some way been inadequate to test the thesis that dietary changes could prevent heart disease. Perhaps they thought the conventional wisdom was so obviously true that it did not require proof.

Whatever the explanation, it is important to note that the negative results of the experiments were entirely consistent with the opinions of many individual doctors and scientists who over the previous fifteen years had argued that fat consumption was *not* a significant cause of heart disease.

Back in 1974, an editorial in the medical journal the *Lancet*, entitled 'Can I Avoid a Heart Attack?' had observed that 'despite all the effort and money that has been spent', the evidence that heart disease was preventable, 'added up to little more than zero', and that 'the only unassailable criterion of preventive success is a reduction in the number of deaths (from heart disease)' – which is exactly what the experiments ten years later failed to provide.[5]

There were other prestigious doubters. In 1977 Professor John McMichael, the mentor of post-war academic medicine in Britain, had written in the *European Journal of Cardiology* : 'It is a sobering thought that our profession has allowed itself to be brainwashed by propaganda into the widespread acceptance of a fashion that can only be transient.'[6] A little while later, Dr George Mann, from Vanderbilt University, was regretting in the pages of the *New England Journal of Medicine* 'the lost generation of misguided and fruitless preoccupation with the diet-heart thesis'.[7] And in 1979 a leading investigator into the science of fat metabolism, Professor E. H. Ahrens from Rockefeller University in New York, contributed a frequently cited article, again to the *Lancet*, concluding that 'dietary recommendations are unwise, impractical and unlikely to lead to a reduced incidence of heart disease'.[8]

For these and other individual scientists, the failure of the

MRFIT and European trials was only too predictable: if food was not an important cause of heart disease, then encouraging people to change their diets would not prevent the disease. So why did the WHO committee not wait for the results of the experiments? At least they could then have given their reasons (if they had reasons) why those results did not influence their proposed solutions. But they did not.

The answer is to be found in the observation that the WHO report was only the first in a whole series of reports from expert committees, all of which asserted the need for radical changes in the Western diet as a preventive measure against heart disease without reference to the results of the tests of those assertions. It began to look as if the public was being sold the beliefs of a group of experts rather than the truth.

In 1983 it was the turn of the British National Advisory Committee on Nutrition Education (NACNE).[9] It, too, reviewed the evidence relating food to disease and came to the same conclusion about the need for radical changes in the nation's diet. But in a dense document complete with graphs, tables and dozens of references, the most recent authority cited in support of its claims turned out to be the WHO committee of the previous year. Once again the trials were not mentioned.

In April 1984 another committee convened a conference, 'Heart Disease Prevention: Plans for Action'. This proposed a 'health promotion team' in each health authority which, by promoting 'dietary and lifestyle' changes in the community, would reduce the death rate from heart disease by 25 per cent. The source of its optimism was undisclosed. The trials were again not mentioned.[10]

Two months later it was the turn of the Department of Health, acknowledging belatedly that the trials had at least taken place: 'They have not shown convincing evidence of benefit', the report observed.[11] But this was only a temporary lapse. During the next three years, three further committees drawn from the same pool of experts purported to examine the scientific evidence. All urged radical changes in the British diet. None mentioned the trials.[12,13,14]

From 1982 to 1987, then, seven different reports argued for major changes in the nation's diet, but six of them found the results of the definitive tests of their claims too embarrassing even to mention. The discrepancy was noted by those in a position to do so. In the midst of these pronouncements, Professor J. R. A. Mitchell, editor of the *International Journal of Cardiology*, observed in 1984:

> To those who keep saying that 'better eating prevents heart disease' we must reply that every evangelist is entitled to his opinion, but every scientist is entitled to ask for the evidence. The claim that the collective beliefs of a prestigious committee can provide a substitute for facts is all too prevalent. . . . We can never be sure of the relationship between the opinions of a committee and the truth.[15]

Those in charge of promoting the campaign, however, were happy to disregard such reservations. Each report naturally attracted considerable publicity – and the constant reiteration of a simple message like the drip of water on stone could not fail to penetrate the consciousness of the public. But the experts were not content to let it rest there. They moved out of their committee rooms into the television studios to hammer the message home; but yet again they failed to acknowledge the evidence contradicting their claims.

In tune with the advice of the 1984 'Plans for Action' conference that the media should 'avoid encouraging confrontation if it leads to confusion', the BBC and commercial stations launched four separate series between 1984 and 1986 promoting the by-now customary message on diet and disease, each replete with images of food and death that omitted any allusion to genuine disagreement or to the scientific experiments in which the value of the proposed dietary changes had been assessed.[16] Perhaps for this reason they proved monotonous.

Opening with a shot of an ambulance screeching through the night or, more gruesomely, a pathologist laying out his tools for a post-mortem, a voice-over intoned chilling statistics about how many people die from certain diseases every year. Then one of the experts would appear to link those diseases to food. Thus, Professor Geoffrey Rose: 'The modern British diet is killing people in their thousands from heart attacks.' (*BBC Food and Health Campaign*); Philip James: 'Diet in my view is the single most important cause of death.' (*World in Action*); and again Geoffrey Rose: 'Modern Western food is the chief cause of our modern epidemic of heart disease.'

There would follow interviews with various protagonists of the diet-disease school, in which every so often a note of caution emerged. Sir Richard Doll: 'There is very little hard evidence, but a reasonable estimate is that perhaps one-third of all fatal cancers are induced by dietary factors.' (*The Food Connection*); and Graham McGregor: 'We don't absolutely know, but we strongly suspect that salt is an important cause of high blood pressure.' (*Food for Thought*). But the overall message was plain, as proclaimed by Philip James: 'The British diet one might describe from the health point of view as one of the most atrocious in the world. There is a whole series of things that are wrong and we have to see a revolution in what we eat.' (*The Food Business*). The programmes side-stepped the scale of the dietary changes decreed by the experts to focus instead on those foods where visual imagery could most powerfully sustain the message – cancer-causing chips, heart-stopping hamburgers.

Then followed a brief visit to a family that had changed over to the new 'healthy diet', and concluding remarks against the backdrop of a cemetery. Geoffrey Rose again:

> Behind each one of these statistics is a personal tragedy, each one has left a home with an empty family, without a breadwinner, a wife without a husband, children without supportive parents. We know enough about the causes of these tragedies and their relation to what we eat – if we could get the scientific information across to the public, then many of these tragedies would be avoided.

As the bandwagon rolled, it gathered momentum and widened its scope. It was not just too much animal fat, but there was an excess of salt and sugar as well. And the Western diet did not just cause heart disease, but strokes, cancers of the bowel and the breast, diabetes, varicose veins, constipation and, most immodestly, piles.

There were many to pick up the message and propagate it further – the Health Education Council, dozens of health education officers, school dietitians and community physicians. Heart disease was, according to John Brown of the HEC, 'the number one killer, and it has been convincingly related to high fat in the diet'. There was not 100 per cent proof that this was the case, but 'by saying nothing we are gambling with people's lives. After all, changes in diet might save tens of thousands of people every year.'

The message provided brilliant copy for the press, which pursued it energetically throughout the country. 'STAFFS CANCER DEATH SHOCK' warned the *Evening Standard* of Stoke-on-Trent: 'Poor cooking and eating habits are to blame for turning North Staffordshire into a cancer black spot.' Community dietitians believed that 'people in this area tend to have a higher than normal level of fat in the diet and it is quite likely this is one of the factors behind the high rate of stomach cancers in the district'. 'A DEADLY DIET' announced the *Northampton Chronicle and Echo* : 'The British are digging their own graves with their teeth', wrote its reporter. 'That is the grim warning of diet experts who believe one in two people endanger their health with the food they eat.' 'WE'RE SO SICK', proclaimed the *South Wales Echo*, interviewing Professor John Catford, the first Professor of Health Education in Europe. The Welsh, he believed, were 'committing nutritional suicide. Mrs Beeton should be thrown in the dustbin.' Later he relented: 'It's all right to have these things sometimes, as long as we eat a frugal diet 90 per cent of the time.'

It is not that easy to get people to change the habits of a lifetime, but institutions can be persuaded. School and hospital canteens cater for a captive audience and where better to start the campaign against food-induced illness? 'Black puddings, fry-ups and fish and chips are facing the chop in Bolton', was the message of the *Evening News* as it outlined the plans of the Royal Infirmary canteen to offer an experimental menu of lentil soup, wholemeal bread and brown rice. The well-intentioned reforms were not universally appreciated: 'Youngsters at Fairfield Hospital are snubbing the new wholesome menu and want chips, fish fingers and sausages', the *Manchester Evening News* reported. The sick children were 'hardly eating anything', but this cut little ice with a health authority spokesman: 'It is our policy to persevere with our healthy eating concept,' he told reporters. 'The children have in different ways highlighted different viewpoints. All they consider is whether they like the food.'

It was the same story in schools. In dozens of classrooms up and down the country children were being educated into the new knowledge of nutrition: fish and chips caused heart attacks, salty crisps caused brain haemorrhages. Ashcombe School in Surrey attached traffic light signals to food in the canteen – red for chips that should be eaten rarely, yellow for iced buns, green for dried bananas. But, 'HANDS OFF OUR CHIPS, SCHOOL BOSSES TOLD', the *South London Press* reported. Tracy Downey (fourteen) told the paper: 'I don't like vegetables or stuff like that. I like curry and rice and sausages.'

At the Christmas buffet dance for hospital staff at Hove Town Hall in 1985, Christmas puddings, pastries, gâteaux, cheese crisps and meat pies were all banned. Instead guests could choose from a variety of pulses, salads and low-fat crisps washed down with a non-alcoholic punch. In Dartmoor the prisoners went on hunger strike in protest at the tasteless low-salt diet inflicted on them by a health-conscious dietitian.

Beyond the health educationalists, the theme was taken up by popular nutritionists in the press. 'The Food that Can Be Fatal' was a typical offering:

> Every time we touch a traditional British fry-up, followed by a mug of tea, we are taking years off our lives. Every bag of sugar, slab of butter, carton of cream, bar of chocolate and pinch of salt should carry a health warning: 'This product may seriously damage your health'.

Most prominent among this group were Geoffrey Cannon and Caroline Walker whose book *The Food Scandal* became a best-seller in 1985.[17] The authors informed readers of *The Times*:

> Leaders of the medical profession now have come to speak of the rate of premature death in this country in apocalyptic terms – as a holocaust, which medicine can do nothing to check. Western food is the main single underlying cause of Western disease.

Cannon and Walker added a new twist to the story by uncovering a conspiracy to suppress the vital information that a change in diet would prevent these illnesses: 'There are some who state from a position of authority that fat, sugar and salt in the quantities consumed in Britain today are harmless to health. As far as I know these people are all employed, paid by or associated with the food industry.' The activity of these sceptics in condoning the food industry's attempts to peddle lethal foodstuffs to the populace was, according to one of Cannon's sources, 'the biggest scandal in British public health since the day 150 years ago when officials refused to act on the fact that cholera and typhoid were caused by open sewers'.

Soon it was time for politicians to exploit the issue. The Labour Party produced a document which its party spokesman Dr Jeremy Bray hoped would bring 'the effect of diet on health to the forefront of political action and debate'. The Junior Tory Health Minister Edwina Currie drew the wrath of northerners by blaming their illnesses on a fondness for chips. And in early 1987 the Conservative Government launched a massive £2 million public health campaign backed by television advertising – 'Look After Your Heart' – in which the central message was the urgent need for changes in the nation's eating habits – a message which emphasised the 'die' in diet.

A continuous line stretches from the WHO committee of 1982, through the media campaign, the health education campaign in schools (the 'diet of death with its holocaust of disease') to its ultimate politicisation. Certainly the content of the argument had shifted away from emphasis on the specific lethal effect of dairy products and meat towards the more acceptable anathematisation of 'junk' foods, but the message remained the same: 'Change your diet and live!'

Yet was any of it true? Medical research had spent many years searching for the causes of these complex illnesses: could it merely be a matter of changing what one had for breakfast? Despite all the pronouncements of the experts from committee rooms and television screens, where was the simple hard evidence that altering the diet would prevent diseases? If there was none (or if, indeed, the evidence suggested the contrary), then surely the public had become the victim of an immense confidence trick?

But there we must leave the British public in the late 1980s. Few could have doubts about the veracity and urgency of the message, but those with long memories might have been a little mystified. They might have recalled that just over fifty years previously equally prestigious and influential expert committees had been producing reports on the role of food in the prevention of disease, but that their recommendations had been the exact opposite of the current wisdom. Rather than cutting down on meat and dairy products, these foods were being vigorously promoted.

In 1936 Sir John Boyd Orr, later Lord Orr, Director of the Food and Agriculture Organization, winner of the Nobel Prize for Peace, had examined the British diet and discovered that for half the population it was deficient in what he called the 'protective constituents' necessary for the 'achievement of optimal health'. He modestly proposed an increase in the consumption of dairy foods – milk, butter and eggs – and meat by one-quarter. The following year the Government trumped these proposals by advising that milk consumption be doubled. And in 1939 the British Medical Association advised that 'to bring the nation's diet up to the optimum', milk consumption should rise by 80 per cent, butter by 40 per cent, eggs by 55 per cent and meat by 30 per cent.[18]

At the same time, probably the best known nutritionist of the day, Sir Robert McCarrison, had been looking at the relationship between food and specific illnesses and found that many infections, intestinal problems, difficulties in pregnancy and childhood neuroses, as well as nephritis (inflammation of the kidneys) and raised blood pressure were caused by deficiencies in the diet of eggs, dairy foods, meat and wholemeal bread.

As these recommendations and discoveries were the exact opposite of our present contemporary wisdom, it is legitimate to ask how doctors and scientists could have generated two absolutely contradictory sets of nutritional proposals within fifty years. In order to answer this question it is necessary to look more closely at the science of nutrition itself.

3
The Mysteries of Nutrition

One of the most remarkable things about nutrition, so commonplace that it is hardly given a thought, is the fact that there is no such thing as an ideal diet. (D. S. McLaren)[1]

The contradictory nutritional advice of the last fifty years has essentially entailed embracing meat and dairy foods as uniquely beneficial and then condemning them as specifically harmful. This would appear to run contrary to common sense: all the different societies of the world have been sustained by different patterns of food consumption which would make it difficult to point to the specific properties (whether beneficial or harmful) of any one type of food. So the validity of the contradictory advice would certainly be considerably clarified if it were possible to reveal the mechanisms which permit humans to flourish in many different nutritional environments.

Nutrition is a sophisticated science. It can describe well the chemical composition of foods, how they are metabolised and excreted. Its medical importance comes in the classical applications of the relation of food to illness, where it has delineated the consequences of over- and under-nutrition, the role of vitamins and minerals in health, and the effects of failing to absorb food. But it is an altogether simpler and more straightforward affair to clarify these effects on health than to try to understand how the body copes with many different patterns of food consumption – how it is that:

Any of the almost infinite variety of diets composed of foodstuffs cultivated locally and consumed in amounts to satisfy hunger has, throughout the entire history of mankind and all over the world, proved capable of meeting all the complex nutritional requirements of Man for normal growth, a healthy life under widely varying conditions, and the successful continuity of the species.[1]

For those brought up in the West, the importance of spiders, grubs and insects in the Indochinese cuisine is perplexing. The Indochinese might well be equally perplexed by the fondness of sections of Western society for high game and decaying cheeses. Yet irrespective of the particular foods used in Indochinese or Western cooking, both cuisines can provide the energy and vital ingredients necessary for healthy life. This means that the human body must be capable of abstracting from the cornucopia of all available foods its own specific requirements; that it must be able to impose the discipline of its own internal needs on the anarchic profusion of the external world.

How is this done? The answers are not clear because the processes involved are as yet too complex for human understanding; but glimpses of what is involved can be found by examining three of them: transformation, self-regulation and adaptation.

Consider first the transformation of the immense chemical spectrum of food that is offered up for human consumption into the building blocks of the human organism. Our requirements from food are quite specific: we must have sufficient calories – that is, enough to eat – and a sufficiency of vitamins, minerals and other essential substances. And we need to be able to obtain these irrespective of whether our main source of food is, as for the vast majority of mankind, a cereal and some vegetables; or whether it is, as for some people, almost entirely of animal origin; or whether, as in the West, there is a choice of 6,000 different foods on the shelves of the average supermarket.

It is easier to understand how formidable the task of transformation is if we think of food-consumption patterns in terms of their basic constituents – fats, carbohydrate and protein. All diets get about 10 per cent of their calories from protein, of either animal or vegetable origin. Beyond this the variation is enormous. Peasant societies consuming a staple cereal with a legume can get up to 85 per cent of their calories from carbohydrate, Western societies about 50 per cent. Societies heavily dependent on animal foods obtain 80 per cent of their calories from fat, while the Hos (an aboriginal tribe in India) derive less than 2 per cent of their calories from that source. But irrespective of the chemical composition of food consumed, it is transformed into the human chemical profile which is the same the world over – 60 per cent water, 18 per cent protein, 15 per cent fat and 1 per cent carbohydrate.

The famous catchphrase 'You are what you eat' thus appears to be the reverse of the truth. A human is remarkably the same being whether brought up on the plains of India or in the urban chaos of New York.

This phenomenon of transformation might be compared to a factory that can take in many different metals in many different forms and widely differing quantities and turn out at the end of the production process one standard, beautifully rolled steel. The corollary of transformation is that it is theoretically unlikely that any one type of food will have a specifically deleterious or beneficial effect on health.

What about self-regulation? One of the myriad of physiological processes in the body illustrates what this involves. Glucose is the energiser of the body's cells: when the level of blood glucose falls (as sometimes happens when a diabetic takes too much insulin) the patient lapses into a potentially lethal coma unless urgently revived with an injection of glucose. Since the dividing line between consciousness and unconsciousness, life and death is a small change in the level of glucose in the blood, it must be vitally important that in everyday life the glucose level stays well within its normal defined limits.

Carbohydrate foods are a major source of glucose, so one might easily assume that everyone needs a constant and steady supply of these foods to sustain the level of blood glucose and thus life. And yet the fact is that even if there is no food at all, even if the body is starved for a month, the level of glucose in the blood will remain constant.[2] How is this achieved?

Stores of glucose in the liver and muscle are slowly released into the bloodstream. Protein is released from muscle and transformed into glucose. Meanwhile the fat stores in the body are mobilised and broken down into free fatty acids and other novel sources of energy that reduce the body's reliance on glucose. The whole is a masterpiece of synchrony and interconnection. And what is true for the self-regulation of glucose applies to the maintenance of constant levels of dozens of other minerals, vitamins, enzymes and hormones in the body.

The obvious consequence of self-regulation is that it is very difficult to influence the functioning of the body by changing one's diet. Self-regulation ensures the maintenance of a 'steady state' of all the physiological variables of the body in the face of radically changing circumstances in the outside world. It is thus fallacious to suggest that people can simply influence for the better the functioning of their body – whether it is the level of glucose or cholesterol in the blood, or their blood pressure – by changing what they eat.

For example, salt is essential to life and involved in many physiological processes. It is found in many foods and used to enhance flavour in cooking. The body will, however, only utilise the amount that it requires. Take too much salt and the body self-regulates by excreting the excess in the urine; take too little salt and it is rigorously conserved by the kidneys.

Excess salt has been incriminated as a cause of raised blood pressure and hence of strokes, and experts have therefore advised its consumption be reduced. But it is possible to influence the blood pressure only by going to extremes of salt intake – consume massive amounts and the blood pressure might rise a little, take hardly any at all and it might fall (or it might not). But between these extremes, self-regulation means that changes in salt intake have little effect on the blood pressure.

The third process to consider is 'adaptability', and this takes us deep into the mysteries of nutrition.

The complex mechanisms of nutrition are not ends in themselves, but means to an end that permits individuals to function in the world. If the external world changes, the body must be able to adapt to those changes. We could not survive if our body were sensitive or vulnerable to sudden changes in the external world, so it *must* be able to adapt.

Now, a fundamental function of food is to provide calories – energy for work and exercise. So what happens if the amount of calories available suddenly changes, if it becomes suddenly possible to eat much more than previously or, as is much commoner, suddenly the amount of food is dramatically reduced?

Major increases in food intake have been investigated many times in the laboratory, where groups of healthy volunteers have been encouraged to overconsume massively. A classic in this field is 'Gluttony: an experimental study of overeating low- or high-protein diets', published in 1967.[3] Eight student volunteers were encouraged to consume in addition to their habitual daily food intake of 2,500 calories, an excess amount of 1,330 calories per day. At the end of the experiment they had each eaten an 'extra' 35,000 calories which should have resulted in an increase in weight of 6 kg. In fact they put on less than one-sixth of this, all in the early days of the study. So what happened to the missing 5 kg? Again the answer is not known, although the leading theory is that there is some mechanism whereby the body 'burns off' excess calories in the form of increased heat production.

At the other extreme, the effects of prolonged food restriction have also been investigated. Here the evidence comes from the experience of civilian prisoners of war in the Far East studied by the Medical Research Council.[4] The conditions in these prison camps were horrendous, the available food falling far below what would normally be considered desirable. Rice, beans and vegetables were the staple, but 'inedible foreign material might reduce the amount by as much as 30 per cent. . . . Weevil infestation of cereals and pulses was very great in the later years.'

The MRC report noted:

> The most interesting period was from May 1943 to September 1944; the total fuel value of the diet showed little variation, remaining around 1,500 calories per day. For eight months there was a steady fall in weight, but after that it ceased to fall and it appeared that a new equilibrium had been reached at a lower metabolic level . . . the body seemed to settle down to a new equilibrium at a body weight 25 per cent less than previously.

At this new equilibrium a considerable though diminished amount of work could be done, certainly sufficient for the prisoners to maintain themselves and essential services by their own efforts. Interestingly, despite severe food restrictions, the overall death rate in these civilian camps was not higher than was normal for the general population in the years before the war.

In this example the adaptability of the body to low energy intakes is particularly conspicuous, but there are whole societies which have adapted to this level of calorie consumption.

Of all the many aspects of nutrition, it might seem possible to advise people how much they should eat; yet not only does that requirement vary from one individual and one society to another, but adaptability demonstrates that the amount of food consumed can change dramatically with astonishingly little subsequent effect on function. As Professor J. V. G. Durnin, from Glasgow University, and colleagues pointed out in a letter to the science journal *Nature*: 'Energy requirements of man and the balance of intake and expenditure are not known.'[5] Not because we don't yet know, but because the variability is so wide and the ability to adapt so sophisticated that it is not possible to put a figure on it. And if it is not possible to place wide limits on the desirable minimum or maximum amount of food that people should consume, what scientific rationale can there be for suggesting that the public should increase or decrease the amount of one specific type of food, such as meat and dairy products?

The effect of the three phenomena of transformation, self-regulation and adaptability is to allow us to survive and prosper in a wide variety of different circumstances and cultures by protecting our internal homeostasis against the vagaries and unpredictability of the natural world. The processes deny the possibility that there can be a straightforward relationship between patterns of food intake and specific diseases. If that is the case, then it is likely that those illnesses which *can* be attributed to food will not arise because people eat one type of food rather than another, such as too many or too few dairy foods, but where the overall pattern of food intake is in some ways exceptional: obesity and starvation will be found at the extremes of over- and under-nutrition; vitamin- and mineral-deficiency syndromes arise in extremely unbalanced diets.

Even with obesity and starvation the relationship to food intake is not straightforward. It is customary to grade obesity into three levels of severity. Mild obesity is a common feature of all societies, and although it may be disapproved of culturally and socially, it does not appear to have any serious consequences for health. Gross obesity is easily recognised in those unfortunate individuals waddling down the High Streets of the world – and their life expectation is low. And in between are the moderately obese, who may appear in good health but are vulnerable to illnesses such as late-onset diabetes and arthritis.

Gross obesity, with its attendant health complications, is rare, and although it is true that the only certain solution for its victims is radically to reduce the amount of food they consume, for most the problem arises from eating too much for their own needs.

The fat do not have to eat more than the thin, and the cause of their obesity remains obscure, though genetic factors are certainly involved, since obesity runs in families. So although severe obesity is an important medical problem it is not necessarily a nutritional one, as it does not arise from overeating *per se*.

Similarly, the plight of the starving children of the world is not solely due to insufficient food. Obviously malnutrition arises from an inadequate and poorly balanced diet and *is* correctable by feeding the right food – but this is by no means the whole story. It also involves a whole interrelated complex of factors such as cash and availability of food; the mother's experience and knowledge in feeding children; the demands on her time from domestic and work responsibilities; the quality of sanitation and water supply; how the baby's food is cooked and the likelihood of its being contaminated; the baby's vulnerability to infection, particularly of the gut, leading to an increased need for food; and the effect of the baby's general health on its appetite.[6]

Put another way, feed one baby in a safe Western environment a given amount of food and it will prosper; but the same amount of food in the Third World may be insufficient to compensate for all the other adverse effects on the child's health. Malnutrition is as much (or indeed more) a social problem as it is a specifically nutritional problem.

The second category of classical nutritional disorders are those in which severely unbalanced diets lead to specific vitamin or mineral deficiency syndromes. Scurvy due to lack of vitamin C is the best known. In the eighteenth century this disease alone seemed sufficient to deny Britain its imperialist dreams.[7] In 1740 the British Admiral George Anson left England with 1,955 men in eight ships to circumnavigate the world. He returned four years later with only one ship, having lost 1,415 of his crew. Early in the voyage his men had fallen rapidly hostage to scurvy, the sick dying in their sodden hammocks. A plague of rats infested the ship, eating away the faces, eyes and limbs of the newly dead and running all over the bodies of the barely living sick in their hammocks, many so paralysed and anaesthetised they were unaware their toes had been gnawed away.

Yet less than thirty years later Captain Cook sailed 60,000 miles around the Antarctic over a period of three years, losing only one man from tuberculosis and three from accidents. The different outcome of the two expeditions was almost entirely attributable to the Scottish physician James Lind, who stressed to Cook the importance of green vegetables as a preventive measure against the deadly scurvy and other vitamin deficiencies. There is no more dramatic example of how a severely unbalanced diet can lead to devastating illness, which in turn can easily and rapidly be corrected or prevented by adding the missing ingredients.

All the vitamin-deficiency syndromes are similar in that they arise in people eating severely unbalanced diets. Beriberi, for instance, is found in countries where polished rice denuded of its thiamin-rich husk is the staple food. Diets with practically no whole milk or butter and limited amounts of fruit and vegetables are deficient in vitamin A, and cause xerophthalmia – a condition in which the conjunctiva of the eye becomes dry, thickened and pigmented, leading to eventual blindness.

These deficiency syndromes are almost unknown in societies of moderate prosperity where there is a range of available foodstuffs, and indeed are rare even among the most impoverished. In the West they are seen only in exceptional circumstances of self-neglect or among individual food faddists pursuing single-mindedly a very restricted diet. An exception to this rule is vitamin D deficiency, leading to rickets, but the incidence of this illness is probably more related to overcrowding and limited exposure to sunlight than to specific dietary deficiency. And where these deficiency syndromes do arise they are easily corrected by feeding a better diet or adding to that diet the missing substances.

There are two further categories of illness in which food is important although neither is due to the types or pattern of food consumed. In food poisoning, food has either become infected with an organism, for example chicken with salmonella, or contains a toxic substance such as the hallucinogen found in toadstools. Food allergy, on the other hand, is an idiosyncratic reaction and almost always occurs in individuals who are genetically sensitive to the external environment, which may include food. Milk can cause childhood eczema, and the colouring tartrazine can cause asthma.

Finally there is a group of illnesses not related to food, but in which a knowledge of nutrition is important for their correct management: diabetics need high-carbohydrate diets, patients with chronic renal failure need low-protein diets.

So in reviewing the relationship of food to disease it is possible to make a generalisation that disease will only arise where the diet – that is, the choice and quantity of foods – is severely restricted; but specific foods, with the exception of the idiosyncratic allergic reactions just mentioned, are not a specific cause of illness, nor indeed a specific cure. This latter is true even for the vitamin deficiency syndromes. Any food that contains vitamin C will cure scurvy – whether it comprises leaves, citrus fruit or potatoes. Only by ignoring the complex physiological processes that underpin nutrition and allow humans to prosper with a wide variety of different diets is it possible to exculpate or incriminate specific foods.

*

But it is exactly this that forms the basis of the contending nutritional wisdoms with which this book is concerned: that meat and dairy foods promoted health in the 1930s, and are a cause of disease in the 1980s – a contradiction that can be neatly summarised in two statements. In 1946 H. E. Magee, a government scientist, described milk as 'the keystone of the nutritional arch', reflecting a widespread nutritional belief of the time.[8]

In 1984 Professor Sir Douglas Black, a former President of the Royal College of Physicians, was quoted in *The Times* as saying 'milk is a killer'.[9] It is hard to conceive of two more strongly

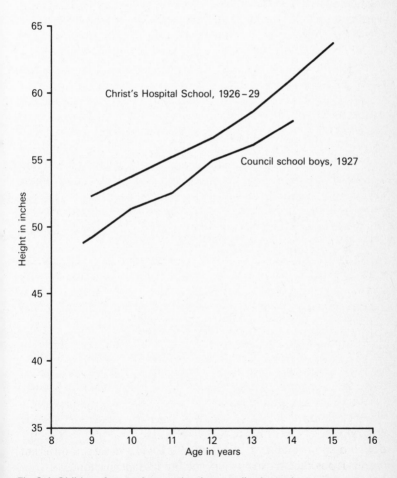

Fig.3.1 *Children from private schools are taller in each age group than those from council schools*

antithetical views and yet zero knowledge of nutrition is needed to know that both are false. There are many societies in which children consume little or no milk at all, but grow up quite obviously healthy. By contrast, the Masai, who take up to 80 per cent of their energy intake as milk, may be equally healthy.

As milk is self evidently neither uniquely beneficial nor specifically lethal the question arises as to what sort of arguments can be deployed to justify first one position and then its opposite. The contradictory views of the health properties of milk are not based on demonstrating its direct beneficence or lethality, but on an inappropriate extrapolation from the valid observation that children who consume a lot of milk will be receiving more calories than those brought up on a carbohydrate-based diet (because fat-based foods contain more calories than the carbohydrate equivalent) and so are likely to grow faster.

Milk is the Keystone of the Nutritional Arch

It had long been noted that there was a height differential between different social classes as shown in a graph contrasting the height of boys from a private school, Christ's Hospital, and their peers at Council schools (Fig. 3.1).[10] In the years between the two World Wars this differential was increasingly attributed to diet and particularly the relatively higher consumption of dairy products by children from the higher social classes. The most powerful evidence in favour of this assumption was a series of feeding experiments conducted by Hugh Corey Mann in the 1920s under the auspices of the Medical Research Council.[11]

Corey Mann took a dismal institution on the outskirts of London and proceeded to show that what had hitherto been considered an adequate diet could be improved by a small supplement of milk. The institution itself evokes the image of a Dickensian world:

> In a great many cases the parentage of the boys is unknown . . . others have recently been rescued as destitute children. Most of the inmates spent all their childhood in the institution until drafted abroad under various emigration schemes or they joined the mercantile marine or Royal Navy.

It was bread, margarine and cocoa for breakfast, bread, margarine and jam for tea. Beef, steamed potatoes and cabbage made Sunday a special day as there was little meat during the week. The diet might have been a penance for the foundlings but it provided a splendid opportunity to test the hypothesis that the height advantage of the socially privileged stemmed from their greater consumption of dairy foods, by giving milk supplements to some of the boys and seeing whether they grew faster than the others.

Over a period of four years the height and weight of the children was monitored on the basic diet and then on experimental diets to which a small additional supplement had been added – either watercress, sugar, New Zealand butter, vegetable margarine or milk. The children who benefited most were those on an extra pint of milk per day: compared to the control group of children, they gained almost twice as much height and weight.

Corey Mann commented:

> Apart from the marked gain in weight and height, there was also a general improvement in their condition, they became far more high spirited and irresponsible, being often in trouble on that account . . . there was however no indication of greater proficiency in school.

The Medical Research Council was very impressed by this study and made the relevant points: 'The unmistakable betterment in nutrition was proved by trial to be due, not to the relatively small increases in the energy provided, nor to the extra protein, but rather to more specific qualities of milk as food.'

If milk had specific growth-enhancing qualities and the government wanted a sturdy, well-grown population, then obviously a move should be taken to ensure that all children received a special quota of milk; this they did with the subsequent introduction of free school milk, which became a central feature of school life for almost fifty years.

So everyone was happy, or almost everyone. The dairy industry was able to dispose of its surplus milk, the Government could feel pleased it was contributing to the health of the nation, nutritionists could feel gratified they had demonstrated the unique virtues of milk. Only the unfortunate minority of children who disliked milk and for whom the mid-morning milk break was something of an ordeal could complain.

However, it will be noted that certain aesthetic and philosophical assumptions lay behind the scientific conclusion that milk was an essential constituent of the diet. Chief among these was the equation of tallness with health.

Tallness is a socially desirable attribute in all societies because of its association with wealth and prosperity, although it is not necessarily desirable for those, like miners, who have to work in confined spaces. But is it necessarily synonymous with health? The question is illuminated by contrasting the views held by nutritionists of the 'genetic potential' school and of the 'functional adaptability' school.

Consider again the contrast between the sons of the affluent at Christ's Hospital and the Council schoolboys. In functional terms both groups are very similar, they have no physical signs of malnutrition, they run around and misbehave and will eventually grow up to be model citizens. However, it is possible that if the Council schoolboys were given the diet of their peers at Christ's they might grow up to be taller, and might thus be said to have fulfilled their 'genetic potential', i.e. grown as tall as their genes will allow. So if health is defined in functional terms both groups are equal, but if it is defined in terms of 'fulfilling genetic potential' one could argue that the Council boys are deprived. Compared to their peers at Christ's, they might be deemed 'chronically malnourished'.

This difference in interpretation is reflected in the current controversy over the extent of malnutrition in the world. If the height of well-nourished First World children is taken to represent optimal fulfilment of genetic potential it is quite easy to show that 80 per cent of Third World Indian children are chronically malnourished as they fail to achieve the height for age of their peers in the West. If, on the other hand, evidence of impairment of function is the criterion of inadequate nourishment the figure for children with specific signs of nutritional deficiency is nearer 2 per cent.

So the belief that milk is the keystone of the nutritional arch is based on several different assumptions: an aesthetic assumption that tallness is intrinsically desirable, and an idealist assumption that everyone should achieve their genetic potential. These are grafted on to two scientific assumptions, that tallness equates with health and that milk as a food has specific growth-enhancing properties. But are these scientific assumptions justified? Where, in particular, is the evidence that children who grow rapidly enjoy a longer or better life than those who grow more slowly? As it is, the belief that milk is a killer is partly based on showing that the disease of breast cancer can be promoted by early rapid growth.

'Milk is a Killer'

The contrary belief that 'milk is a killer' is based on linking the diseases of Western society with the Western diet, which, being high in dairy products and meat, has a relatively high fat content. The evidence to support the belief comes from cross-cultural studies in which differing patterns of disease in different countries are compared with dietary patterns.

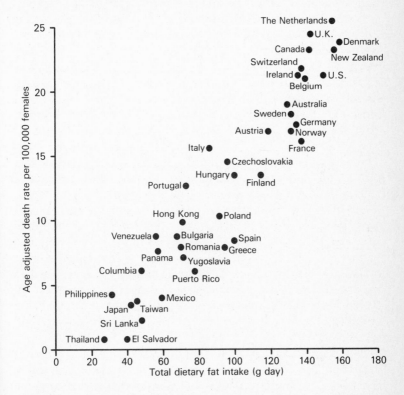

Fig.3.2 *The mortality rate from breast cancer in different countries is strongly related to the amount of fat in the diet*

One of the most convincing of these relationships is the incidence in different countries of breast cancer, which increases markedly with the amount of fat in the diet (Fig. 3.2).[12] The deduction which might be drawn is that fat has specific cancer-inducing properties, and that were people to reduce their consumption of dairy foods they would reduce their risk of breast cancer. Before accepting this prescription it is as well to find out a bit more about breast cancer.[13]

Breast cancer is a hormone-dependent cancer – that is, its growth is facilitated by the female hormones, and the disease can be checked by giving drugs that block the actions of those hormones. It is not surprising, therefore, that the risk of the disease depends on the length of time the breast is exposed to those hormones from puberty to the menopause, i.e. the length of the 'reproductive life.' The longer the duration of reproductive life, the longer the breast is exposed to hormones and the higher the risk of breast cancer.

The initiating mechanism of puberty remains obscure, but it seems to be related to rate of growth, which in turn is related to social status and general health, such as exposure to infections and diet. Girls living in Western societies with a high standard of public health and a lot of dairy produce in the diet grow quickly (because dairy foods contain a lot of calories); they have an early puberty and will have a late menopause; and so they have a higher risk of breast cancer compared to girls from other societies. Another influence on breast cancer is the age of first pregnancy; if this is delayed, as it frequently is in the West, it also increases risk of the disease.

Thus the relationship between fat consumption and breast cancer is indirect, a reflection of the impact of a type of diet on growth rates, and of a cultural tendency to delay the first pregnancy. The corollary is that adult women have no hope of influencing their own risk of the disease by changing their dietary pattern; but if parents could change their daughters' lives drastically enough to take them back down the path of development, alter their diet sufficiently to slow down early growth, curtail their reproductive lives and also encourage them to conceive earlier, then their risk of the disease might fall.

So in reviewing the contradictory perceptions of the role of milk in health, the consideration is really the effect on growth rates. If one chooses tallness as a desirable attribute, equates this with health, shows that it can be increased with milk supplements, describes milk as a 'protective food', then milk does become the 'keystone of the nutritional arch'. But if one focuses on breast cancer and shows that its incidence between different countries rises with increasing consumption of fat; misinterprets that observation as indicating that fat consumption is a direct cause of breast cancer, rather than that it exerts this effect by promoting rapid early growth, an early puberty and prolonged reproductive life; incriminates milk as contributing to that fat consumption; and describes it not as a protective food but under the pejorative heading of 'saturated fat', then milk becomes a 'killer'.

It so happens that the example of breast cancer provides much the strongest evidence of a disease that is (albeit only indirectly) associated with a specific type of food. But it is time now to turn back to the 1930s, when it was inconceivable that meat and dairy foods could be considered harmful, when a diet could not be regarded as healthy unless it contained them in abundance.

4
The Healthy Diet of 1936

Britain between the wars produces two contrasting images. For some it was 'The Long Weekend'. In Evelyn Waugh's writings the young danced.

> What a lot of parties (masked parties, Greek parties, Wild West parties, Russian parties, parties where one had to dress as someone else, almost naked parties in St John's Wood, parties in flats and studios and shops and hotels and night clubs and swimming baths).[1]

And yet the image that persists is George Orwell's much more sombre one:

> At the back of one of the houses, a young woman was kneeling on the stones, poking a stick up the leaden pipe which I suppose was blocked. I had time to see everything about her – her seedy apron, her clumsy clogs, her arms reddened by the cold. She looked up as the train passed, and I was almost near enough to catch her eye. She had a round pale face, the usual exhausted face of the slum dweller who is 25 and looks 50, thanks to miscarriages and drudgery, and it wore for the second in which I saw it, the most desolate, hopeless expression I have ever seen.[2]

The strong contrast of a divided Britain dominated political perceptions. The Left saw only decay, the final working out of the 'contradictions of Capitalism'. Orwell's kneeling woman conscious of her oppression would, under the leadership of a revolutionary party, usher in a new golden age. In the words of Harry Pollitt, head of the Communist Party: 'The stark reality is that for the mass of the population, Britain is a hungry Britain, badly fed, clothed and housed.'[3]

Subsequent historians have been less than sympathetic to this interpretation of events. The 'hungry thirties' was a 'myth sedulously propagated'.[4]

The Right saw in the depression of the 1930s an aberration of an economic system that had served them well for two centuries. Euphemism concealed the problems of poverty and unemployment; those hardest hit were confined to the 'distressed areas', and their experience had little universal significance.

Against this background of political conflict, on 8 July 1936, the House of Commons met to debate a motion put forward by the Labour MP Thomas Johnston: 'This House has noted the growing evidence of widespread malnutrition . . . and regrets the continued failure of His Majesty's Government to take effective steps to deal with the grave and unjust problem of hunger and want in the midst of plenty.'[5] Nutrition had moved centre stage into the political arena, throwing its weight behind the forces of social discontent. Its impact was enormous.

Foremost among the scientific authorities called on by the motion's proposer were Sir John Boyd Orr, who had shown that '9 million people in the country had a diet defective in protective constituents', and Sir Robert McCarrison, who had recently claimed in a prestigious public lecture that the figure for malnourishment among children was 'several times the official figures'.

The malnutrition question was to be debated many times in the coming years. Time and again these scientific authorities were summoned to support the Opposition's case. The indictment of the political system ceased to be merely the predictable polemics of the Left and its allies, but had been confirmed by an important section of the scientific community. What was the objective scientific evidence that Boyd Orr and McCarrison had discovered and the Left found so convincing?

In the early part of 1936, Sir John Boyd Orr had published *Food, Health and Income*, in which he sought to define a state of 'optimum nutrition – a state of well being such that no improvement can be effected by a change in diet'.[6]

The study started by assessing the food intakes of different classes in society, analysed them in terms of their basic constituents, and compared the results with a set of Recommended Daily Allowances (or RDAs) that had been drawn up by nutritionists over the previous decade. It was then possible to determine the percentage of the population who were in a state of 'optimal' nutrition, that is above the RDA level, and those with a 'suboptimal' level of nutrition, that is below the RDA level.

The central part of Boyd Orr's survey was an analysis of the consumption patterns of 1,152 families subdivided into six 'classes' according to the average expenditure per head of each family ranging from 4 shillings in group 1 to 14 shillings in group 6. (This is the opposite of the current Registrar-General's classification of social class that has group 1 at the top with the highest disposable income and group 5 at the bottom with the lowest.)

As would be expected, the consumption of staple foods – bread, flour and potatoes – varied little between the classes, but that of more expensive foods – fresh milk, butter, meat and fruit – varied enormously, with an up to fourfold difference in consumption. Predictable too were the foods – condensed milk and margarine – in which the trend was reversed with a much higher consumption among the less well-off.

The next step was to convert the different patterns of food consumption between the classes into the amounts of specific nutrients in the diet and see how they compared with the Recommended Daily Allowances. When this was done Boyd Orr was able to demonstrate that the diet of the social group with the lowest income (group 1) was deficient in virtually every important constituent including calcium, iron and vitamin C, and also that they were not getting enough to eat. Those in the intermediate income class (group 3) were apparently obtaining sufficient calories, but were below standard for minerals and vitamins, and only among the wealthy (group 6) were 'the standard requirements met in every case'.

Applying these observations to the whole nation, he was thus able to demonstrate that the diet of half the population was deficient in 'protective constituents' (i.e. those elements that were meant to protect against disease), an observation that was interpreted by politicians and the public as indicating that there was widespread malnourishment especially among the poorer classes. This section of the report does however end with a disclaimer:

> It should be kept in view that the standards with which the above comparisons are made are those compiled for the maintenance of perfect health. . . . . These diets may be sufficient to maintain life and a certain degree of activity and yet be inadequate for the maintenance of the fullest degree of health which a perfectly adequate diet would make possible.

To raise the standard of nutrition that would be adequate for the maintenance of the 'fullest degree of health' with sufficient 'protective constituent' would require an increase in consumption of milk, dairy products, eggs and meat by one-quarter.

The survey did not attempt to identify directly any who might have definite signs of malnourishment but relied instead on the height differential between the upper-class boys from Christ's Hospital and those from Council schools (encountered in Chapter 3) as evidence that the differences in dietary patterns were significant:

> These differences in height are in accordance with what would be expected from an examination of the diets in common use in these classes. In the lower income groups, the diet is relatively deficient in the constituents required for growth. Too high a proportion of the diet comes from carbohydrate-rich foods which contain very little bone- and flesh-forming material.

The second scientific authority invoked by the politicians concerned with the problem of malnutrition was Sir Robert McCarrison, who took a different but complementary position to that of Boyd Orr. Rather than determining the extent of malnutrition, he argued in a series of prestigious public lectures during 1936 that most diseases were due to a 'faulty' diet.[7]

McCarrison had spent a lifetime as colonial medical officer in India and had been forcibly impressed by the apparent differences in health of the races of that country. This had led him to the belief that:

> The greatest single factor in the acquisition and maintenance of good health is perfectly constituted food. No other factor, neither race nor climate, nor endemic disease has so profound an influence as food in determining the levels of physical efficiency among the Indian races.

The races of southern India, with little in the way of dairy foods, were of poor physique and vulnerable to many more diseases than their chappatti-eating, milk-drinking northern neighbours – the Sikhs. As a consequence he believed they were much more prone to tuberculosis, leprosy, dysentery, duodenal ulcers, rheumatism, cancer, mental diseases and many others.

While in India he had conducted a series of experiments, feeding laboratory rats on the wide variety of diets of the Indian peoples, from the Sikhs in the north to the Madrassis in the south. Whereas those on the Sikh diet prospered, those on the Madrassi diet showed 'stunted growth and other signs of poor condition'. These results, he believed:

> confirmed the observations made on man himself . . . the best diet that of the Sikhs contained an abundance of every element and complex needed for normal nutrition . . . the worst that of the Madrassis was excessively rich in carbohydrate and deficient in suitable protein.

He subsequently turned his attention to the poorer classes in Britain, feeding his rats on what he estimated to be their typical diet, 'white bread, margarine, over-sweetened tea and little milk, boiled potatoes and tinned meat'. These animals showed similar signs to the rats fed on the Madrassi diet. Of course the two diets were very different, but it was their 'imperfect constitution' that was responsible for illness.

Later in 1936 McCarrison enlarged on this theme in a further lecture to the British Medical Association in Oxford, in which he was to attribute most diseases to food.[8] The 'newer knowledge of nutrition' had, he claimed, revealed the following sequence of events: 'faulty food, faulty nutrition, faulty function, faulty health, disease'. So the imperfectly constituted diet increased susceptibility to infection and major gastrointestinal disease; in obstetrics it led to habitual abortion, prolonged gestation and uterine bleeding; and it also led to most of the neuroses of childhood, especially headaches, to insomnia, and to a multitude of others, including 'typhoid fever, nephritis, raised blood-pressure, diabetes, chronic arthritis, even tuberculosis'. All these conditions, he argued, could be treated by instituting nutritional changes based on 'the fundamental principles of the correction of food faults'.

McCarrison was imprecise as to the exact mechanism by which faulty diet was responsible for all these ailments, but suggested it might be due to 'suboptimal' amounts of essential vitamins and minerals in the diet. He felt on firmer ground in recommending foods which when 'properly combined in the diet are known to constitute perfect nutrition, a good whole cereal grain, milk and its products, butter and cheese, eggs, fruit and meat'.

He was particularly emphatic about the virtues of brown wholemeal bread over the white 'refined' product, reflecting the contemporary opinion that refining flour was a harmful nutritional practice because it stripped this basic food of its life-enhancing vitamins.

Boyd Orr and McCarrison were certainly not alone in claiming that malnourishment and faulty nutrition were widespread and the cause of much avoidable illness, although their views were disputed by a few contemporary doctors and scientists – to little avail. For the moment it is only necessary to try to understand the basis for the plausibility, and widespread acceptance, of their authority on these issues.

Intrinsic to the characterisation of the defects of the British diet was the concept that some foods (meat and dairy products) were intrinsically superior to others (white bread and potatoes), that they had more protective constituents, more health-enhancing properties. The basis for this lay in the discovery over the preceding half-century that there were indeed vital constituents of food – the vitamins – whose absence in severely restricted or unbalanced diets did indeed lead to a variety of illnesses, the vitamin-deficiency syndromes.

The potency of these discoveries in influencing medical thought into the belief that types of food consumed were an important and remediable cause of illness can best be demonstrated by considering two of them in more detail: beriberi and rickets.

The emphasis on the virtues of unrefined brown bread arose from the discovery that refining another cereal – rice – that is, removing its vitamin-containing husk led to the vitamin-deficiency syndrome beriberi. Dairy foods more obviously were to be commended because they contained a substance, vitamin D, that prevented against the disease rickets.

There are two types of the exotically named beriberi: 'wet' beriberi in which the patient retains fluid, becoming swollen and oedematous; and 'dry' beriberi which attacks the nerves of the legs, leading to paralysis. Both are caused by a deficiency of thiamin or vitamin B. It is classically a disease of the rice-eating communities in the Far East, particularly those who eat 'polished' rice from which the thiamin-containing rice rusk or germ has been removed by milling. In 1883 a Dutchman Christian Eijkmann was sent by his government to Java with specific instructions to find the bacterium responsible for the disease.[9]

The belief that beriberi was caused by a bacterium was predictable, for this was the time when Pasteur, Koch and many other scientists in Europe were revealing microscopic disease-causing bacteria to an astonished world.

> With the work of Pasteur and Koch . . . there penetrated into all
> fields of medicine the idea that infinitely small bugs endowed with
> specific pathogenic properties played a pre-eminent role in pro-
> ducing many diseases. The new concept made such an impression
> that for a while it was believed that the cause of all diseases could
> be ascribed to microbes alone . . . almost completely dominant,
> bacteriology at this period became the centre and goal of medical
> investigation.[10]

If the bacterium responsible for a disease had not as yet been
identified, that was only because people had not looked hard
enough. And that was Eijkmann's mission.

Bacteriological work relied on experimenting with animals, and
Eijkmann used chickens. His initial observation that led him to
suppose that beriberi might be a nutritional rather than a bacteriological disease owed much to chance.

> His original research in beriberi began in a curiously accidental
> way. He wished to carry out certain investigations on fowls, and
> in order to economise on their food he fed them on scraps from
> the wards of the military hospital to which he was attached. On
> these scraps which consisted chiefly of cooked polished rice the
> fowls developed paralysis, whose nature was at first obscure. A
> clue thereto was unintentionally given by a newly appointed
> director of the hospital, who refused to let Eijkmann feed his
> fowls any longer on scraps from the wards. Henceforth they
> were fed on gaba (rice still in the husks) and on this diet they
> recovered.[11]

There are many causes of paralysis and it was only a hunch that
the condition induced in chickens was the same beriberi that he
had been sent out to investigate. But it was a hunch he decided to
pursue. Other bacteriologists also looking for a bacterium as the
cause of the disease found them in abundance. Glockner identified
an amoeba, Fhaardo a haematozoon, Pereira a spherical micro-
organism, Durham a looped streptococcus, Taylor a spirillum,
Winkler a staphylococcus and Dangerfield an aerobic micrococcus.
There were many others.

Eijkmann had a colleague in the civil medical inspectorate in Java
with whom he collaborated in conducting a survey into the health of
prisoners on the island. The results were astonishing: 'Of nearly
300,000 prisoners, only 1 in 10,000 of those who ate unpolished rice
had beriberi, whereas 1 in 39 who ate polished rice suffered from the
disease.' Certain that the husk of the rice germ contained the secret

of his mission, Eijkmann was able, with crude biochemical techniques, to extract a substance from the rice germ that protected against the disease a substance to be identified much later as the vitamin thiamin. Subsequent studies in a mental asylum in Kuala Lumpur in which the inmates were fed either polished or boiled rice confirmed that feeding humans polished rice caused the disease.[12]

The discovery of all the major vitamins followed a similar pattern to that of thiamin. Rare diseases in groups of people with unusual or severely unbalanced diets would be replicated in animals fed similarly unbalanced diets. Chemical analyses would later identify a specific missing factor which when given to the victims would cure the disease. In 1911 Casimir Funk brought together all these strands of investigation in his classic book *The Aetiology of the Deficiency Diseases*, and coined the term 'vitamine' (later to be changed to 'vitamin').

However, as far as the Western world was concerned, diseases specifically attributable to vitamin deficiency were rare indeed, leading many to believe that although the science of the vitamins might be fascinating, they had little relevance to the practice of medicine; then came the discovery of the role of vitamin D in the prevention of rickets.

The name of the disease is derived from the Anglo-Saxon word *wriklen* – to twist. It is caused by a deficiency of vitamin D, which when present in adequate amounts facilitates the absorption of calcium from the gut and the deposition of calcium in bone. Children with the disease have soft bones which, when they start to walk, become deformed, leading to a characteristic bowing of the legs. They can also develop curvature of the spine and deformities of the pelvic bones, which in women leads to obstructed labour in childbirth.

One of the first tasks of the Medical Research Committee after its formation in 1913 was to ask the distinguished scientist Edward Mellanby to investigate the cause of rickets. Reviewing the many theories of the cause of the disease, including the possibility that it was due to an as yet undiscovered infectious agent, Mellanby chose rather to focus on the fact that a diet rich in carbohydrate and poor in animal fat produced faulty bone formation. In a long series of trials in puppies he showed that the disease could indeed be induced with a diet made up predominantly of cereals and that it could be prevented or cured by the addition of fat to the diet. However, the type of fat was important. Vegetable oils were not effective, but cod-liver oil, eggs and dairy products were. Thus there was likely to be a vitamin in these foods that was important in the disease.[13]

But that was by no means the whole story. At the same time, doctors in Glasgow had also been looking for a cause. They fed two groups of puppies on the same diet, keeping one lot in the laboratory, the other in the countryside where they were exercised regularly. Only the laboratory animals developed rickets.[14] And so arose an important controversy – was rickets a dietary disease or was it due to lack of fresh air and exercise? The contending theories seemed to have so little in common that it seemed reasonable to suppose they could not both be right. Conveniently, after the First World War Europe provided an ideal situation in which to resolve the dispute. It was not to be the only time that the distress of children in the aftermath of war would clarify crucial issues of nutrition.

In a large foundling hospital in Vienna, Dr Henrietta Chick and her colleagues from the Medical Research Council found many young children who had been severely affected by the deprivations of the war years.[15] Their growth, height and general physical development were considerably below what would be considered normal for their age. Many had rickets. The leading medical physicians in Vienna were sceptical that this was due to dietary deficiency. This is illustrated by the opinions of the head of the clinic in which the experiment was to be conducted, Professor Clemens von Pirquet:

> When Dr Chick and her colleagues began their work in 1919 I had little expectation that it would lead to results of much practical value. At this time I was of the opinion that vitamin deficiency was a very rare occurrence. As for rickets I held the view that it was an infectious disease producing severe symptoms only in those who possessed special susceptibility. . . . I believed that the more severe symptoms of rickets were shown first by children who became infected shortly after birth, that is to say infants who in the overcrowded dwellings of the proletariat class, came into contact with other cases of rickets at an early age.

Dr Chick sought the answers to two questions: what diet prevented rickets and what could be done to treat the disease once it had developed? To answer the first question she took seventy-five apparently healthy children and divided them into two groups, one to receive a standard diet the other to receive a diet supplemented by full-cream dried milk and cod-liver oil. The first and most striking finding was that none of the children developed rickets during the summer months, but in the winter months from October to May fourteen of twenty-four children not receiving the milk and cod-liver oil developed the disease. This finding was compatible with the dietary theory but also with that of the Glaswegian doctors who had proposed the environmental explanation of a relative lack of exposure to fresh air and sunlight.

When it came to treating rickets once it had developed, the investigators tried three options: some received cod-liver oil supplements, others were exposed to ultraviolet light and a third group received sunlight only. Each method of treatment was effective. So it looked as if both theories of the nature of the disease were correct. The idea that sunlight was important had in fact been postulated as far back as 1890 when a study of the geographical distribution of the disease had shown that its incidence was inversely related to sunlight, so that children in the tropics, despite consuming few dairy foods, also escaped the disease.

How to fit all these findings together? There was an element in the diet, subsequently identified as vitamin D, found in high concentration in dairy foods and cod-liver oil, that protected against the disease in the winter months but was not essential in the summer. In addition there was also a substance in the skin that under the influence of radiation from the sun was transformed into the vitamin. So rickets was commonest in children on poor diets in industrial cities of northern Europe where the natural lack of sunlight was compounded by the smoky atmosphere and a diet with few dairy foods. It was rare in children eating diets with plentiful access to these foods and who had the opportunities to live and play in fresh air.

Vitamin D was eventually characterised and synthesised in 1931. It is now estimated that 90 per cent of the body's vitamin D comes from the action of sunlight on the skin, and a mere 10 per cent from the diet. However, in the 1920s the importance of the body's own source of vitamin D was neglected in favour of emphasis on the importance of the dietary contribution with, as will be seen, ultimately disastrous consequences.

The discovery of the role of vitamin D in the prevention of rickets came at an important moment in the history of medicine. By the early 1920s the germ theory of disease was in decline; not that its contributions to the understanding of disease was no longer important, but most of the significant bacteria that caused disease in humans had already been discovered. Yet the cause of much illness still remained unexplained. Perhaps the answer lay in nutrition? As an idea it had a lot going for it.

Vitamin-deficiency syndromes were certainly rare in the Western world, but possibly there was a level above frank deficiency, 'suboptimal vitamin deficiency', in which the body was not receiving quite the right amount of these magic substances. Perhaps this was important? Only a limited number of vitamins had been discovered; maybe there were many more still to be discovered? And then there was another possibility that 'good nutrition' might protect the body against certain illnesses.

These concepts might be vague, but they held the promise that if science could only identify the best type of diet and ensure that everyone partook of it, this might have a significant impact on disease. In this way nutritional science could be seen as the reverse of the germ theory. The microbe hunters had identified many organisms causing serious disease in humans, but could do nothing about it. Nutrition was uncertain about the specific role of food in disease but offered in the 'ideal diet' an opportunity to exert a major beneficial influence on the pattern of disease.

Nevertheless, it was not until the mid-1930s that recognition of the role of vitamins in health became transformed into the belief that meat and dairy foods had a crucial role in the prevention of illness in Britain, as expressed in the work of Boyd Orr and McCarrison. So what happened during the intervening period to convert interesting scientific discoveries into the basis of an indictment of society?

The answer lies in examining more closely two medical pre-occupations of the time arising from the discovery of the causes of beriberi and rickets – the unique health-giving properties of milk, the nutritional superiority of brown over white bread.

The discovery of the role of dairy products in the prevention of rickets was central to their endorsement as 'protective foods' because they 'protected' against disease. If their deficiency in the diet resulted in bone deformities, then a high dairy-food intake would promote growth and strength of children. This inspired the feeding experiments conducted by Corey Mann (discussed in Chapter 3) which showed that supplementing the diet of institutional children with milk promoted more rapid growth. The results certainly impressed Boyd Orr, who sought further evidence to substantiate the virtues of dairy foods by comparing the physique and health of the African tribe famous for their high consumption of milk, the

Masai, with that of a non-dairy-consuming neighbouring tribe, the Kikuyu.[16]

The Kikuyu had two chief meals: a thick porridge of which the main ingredients were maize, legumes and plantains, and a gruel made from millet flour and water. The Masai were sustained by a diet made up almost entirely of meat, milk and the blood of their cattle. In nutritional terminology, the Kikuyu had a low-fat/high-fibre diet, and the Masai a high-fat/low-fibre diet.

Boyd Orr found that by the age of twenty, the high-fat/low-fibre-eating Masai were 5 inches taller, 27 pounds heavier and 50 per cent stronger (measured by a 'dynamometer') than their Kikuyu peers. He commented in his report:

> The striking difference between the Masai and the Kikuyu raises the question to what extent diet can affect the status and physique of a race. . . . We are probably justified in concluding that the diet commonly in use among the Kikuyu and other tribes of similar customs is badly balanced, being too rich in carbohydrate and deficient in calcium. It is probably deficient also in other substances required as construction material for growth and certain vitamins.

These studies convinced Boyd Orr that the impoverished children at the heart of the Empire needed all the surplus milk that was at that time being poured down the streams and sewers. Under his influence an old colleague who subsequently turned MP, Walter Elliot, introduced a bill through Parliament in 1933 which enabled local authorities to provide free milk for school children.

The final episode in the endorsement of dairy foods was the major study, *Food, Health and Income*, with its apparent demonstration that half the population of the British Isles were malnourished because the lower social classes consumed less meat and dairy foods than their betters.

The case for milk as an indispensable food for growing children was mirrored in the other passionate belief of the time – the nutritional advantage of brown over white bread. White bread was markedly inferior because it lacked the all-important vitamin thiamin, which was removed with the germ at milling. The fact that no cases of beriberi had been seen in Britain, where eaters of white bread obtained their thiamin from other sources, was irrelevant; the mere action of stripping a staple food of such a vital nutritional component was an outrage against good nutritional practice.

The argument over the relative merits of brown and white bread goes back to antiquity and illustrates beautifully the many cultural and psychological influences on what is perceived as healthy eating. In the Middle Ages white bread signified class: 'To have white bread on the table every day was a sign of wealth, and as such gradually became one of the objectives of the poor, especially the city poor and servant class.'[17] And it was important for health: 'the finest white bread was very profitable for the thin, weak, loose and extenuated bodies, but not so commendable for those that are strong', whereas the coarse wheaten loaf was 'wholesome enough, it nauseateth less – but for those that are healthy, and also for such as would not wax gross, it is most profitable.'[18]

There are three interesting ideas here. The whitest flour was best for the 'weak and extenuated' because, having dispensed with the presumed unnecessary wheat germ, it had the most 'concentrated' nutrients. Secondly, however, if one was healthy, it made little difference which type of bread was preferred. Thirdly, white bread was more fattening – presumably because those who ate it were the most prosperous and therefore the plumpest.

A change in the tenor of the argument came in the nineteenth century, associated with the names of two men, Graham and Allinson, who together made 'a deep impression on all those who had any interest in diet and health'. For Graham: 'It is for a wise purpose that the Deity has so intimately associated in the germ the several substances which are necessary for the complete nutrition of animal bodies . . . how unwise we are in attempting to undo this natural allocation of materials.'[19] And Allinson: 'The true staff of life is wholemeal bread, and it is a true staff, one which will not break.'[20] Their belief in the dangers of refining flour invoked powerful imagery of goodness, wholeness and the needs of 'natural man'.

There was, however, an important scientific issue, which the enthusiastic Victorian scientists pursued with vigour: was brown really healthier than white? The initial tide of opinion favoured the white bread protagonists because it appeared to be better absorbed:

> It is often concluded that wholemeal is preferable to white bread because it is richer in protein and mineral matter and so makes for a better balanced diet. But our examinations have shown even if this were the case, the lesser absorption of wholemeal bread would tend to annul the advantage.[21]

But in the early decades of the twentieth century the discovery of the role of vitamins in the prevention of disease finally ensured victory for the protagonists of brown bread. Granted that white bread might be better absorbed, but the removal of the germ stripped bread of its vital vitamin content and who was to know what serious harm might result? All or as many ailments as one wished could be ascribed to this national impoverishment of the diet: cardiovascular disease, retardation of growth, anorexia, diarrhoea and even 'the decline in the birth rate'.

Reviewing the controversy in 1939, the *British Medical Journal* said: 'It might be thought that the battle between brown and white bread has been fought too often and that the recurring victories of the former would justify the cancellation of what has now become a regular fixture.' This did not, however, inhibit it from reiterating the evidence that 'fully confirmed the really serious inferiority of white bread as compared with wholemeal in every criteria of nutritional value so far adopted'.[22]

Two years later, when the exigencies of wartime required the Government to introduce a standard national wholemeal loaf made of unrefined flour, the *Lancet* greeted the decision in a glowing editorial:

> There has been a suspicion in more than one quarter that the interests of the millers have been allowed to stand in the way of the nation's health, and until this moment the Ministry of Food has shown signs of falling short of wholehearted advocacy of the wholemeal loaf. . . . All the evidence goes to show that the human gut rebels against refined foodstuffs and that in eating a quantity of refined foods people do indeed dig their graves with their teeth. It is a punishable offence to water milk and dilute the solids in it. Why then should it be thought praiseworthy to remove from the wheat berry the valuable minerals and vitamins it contains.[23]

In the case for milk and brown bread one sees how it is possible to extrapolate from important but limited scientific discoveries to the attribution of profound powers to specific foods in the promotion of health. Logically, the relative paucity of these foods in the diet of the working class and unemployed was a cause of weakness and illness. But that relative paucity arose from economic inequalities, so these medical problems really belonged in the political arena. Again and again nutrition dominated the political agenda in Parliamentary debates.

On 11 November 1936, a Labour MP claimed that 'in the UK the diet of at least 50 per cent of the population falls short of the desirable standard', and another that there were tens of thousands of children who 'had hardly sufficient strength to break the skin of a rice pudding'. For Alf Greenwood the existence of widespread malnutrition made it a matter of regret that the Government 'had no proposals for making the fundamental changes in the basis of society in order to create a socialist commonwealth to which the full resources of the nation could be utilized for the benefit of the community as a whole'. On 5 May 1937 Viscount Astor accused those medical officers of health who denied the existence of widespread malnutrition as being 'out of date and not acquainted with the new findings of science'.[24]

Against this onslaught the Government made a poor showing. How could they deny there was a problem when distinguished men of science had proved its existence? They were forced back to pointing out that the obvious improvements in the nation's health since the end of the First World War made it unlikely there was a serious nutritional problem in the country. Seven years had been added to the mean expectancy of life; the infant mortality rate had fallen dramatically from 100 to 57 per thousand. And the Government's own medical officers found a major discrepancy between the claims of Boyd Orr and their own perceptions. They were 'hard pressed to find any convincing evidence of malnutrition'. An inspection of 1½ million children carried out in 1935 found that only 0.7 per cent were in poor physical condition.[25] So who was right?

The discovery of the vitamins that inspired the nutritional beliefs of the 1930s were based on the discriminating power of science. As has been seen, the question of whether beriberi was a nutritional or infectious disease, or the relative contribution of food and sunlight in the prevention of rickets, had been resolved by scientists testing the hypothesis: if *a* causes *b*, then changing *a* should change *b*. If polished rice causes beriberi, then unpolished rice should cure it. If rickets is due to a lack of vitamin D in the diet or lack of sunlight, then a diet rich in vitamin D or exposing children to sunlight should cure it. So before re-examining the validity of Boyd Orr and McCarrison's certainties, it is appropriate to look around and see if they too can be tested experimentally. Boyd Orr argued that a major increase in the consumption of meat and dairy products would improve the health of the nation. What would happen if everyone had to eat fewer dairy products? If Boyd Orr was right, their health would deteriorate. If wrong, it would not. As for McCarrison, with his belief in the virtues of wholemeal bread, what would happen if one fed two groups of children a diet consisting mostly of white or brown bread? If white was seriously nutritionally inferior, this would show up in their growth rates and general health.

Both these experiments were conducted over the next fifteen years. From 1939 to 1945 wartime rationing drastically reduced the fat consumption of the British people. In 1947 experiments in a German orphanage finally resolved the white–brown bread argument.

5

Words Without Knowledge

A food policy was critical to Britain's survival in the early years of the Second World War when the forces of Fascism on mainland Europe were attempting to starve the country into surrender. It had two objectives – to ensure self-sufficiency, and through a system of rationing to ensure an equitable distribution of what food there was. The obvious priority was to ensure that everyone had enough to eat – that is, enough calories. As animals can never produce the amount of food equal in calorific value to the crops that might be grown in the same area, extensive tracts of land that previously would have supported dairy cattle, pigs and sheep, were ploughed up for wheat, potatoes and other vegetables, thus increasing the amount of calories available from domestic production by 30 per cent.[1]

That meant that foods of animal origin – eggs, butter, cheese, poultry and all types of meat – had to be rationed along with other luxuries, of which tea was a much regretted casualty. The amount of food available on ration each week was the equivalent of what the average citizen might have consumed in a day in peacetime and ration-day, not surprisingly, displaced pay-day as the most important event in the weekly calendar. The major exception to the decline in meat- and dairy-based food was an increase in the quantities of liquid milk, which was directed mostly towards children and nursing mothers.

A secondary objective of the policy was to ensure that what food was available was as full of desirable nutrients as possible. So flour was 'unrefined', producing in the 'war loaf' a staple food which was considered by experts to be highly desirable on health grounds, but was almost universally disliked. To the loaf was added calcium 'for growing bones' and thiamin just in case anybody might succumb to beriberi. Margarine was fortified with vitamin D, and blackcurrants were promoted as a rich source of vitamin C.

The overall change in food consumption patterns compared to the pre-war years looked like this:

Up

potatoes	45%
vegetables	33%
milk	28%
grain	17%

Down

citrus fruits	50%
other fruits	44%
poultry/fish	39%
fats and oils	16%
meat	21%
eggs	6%

In practical terms, the diet became much heavier and duller, as the loss of the much-prized, tasty animal-based foods had to be made up with larger quantities of (unrationed) cereal and vegetables. The significant issue as far as the pre-war nutritional recommendations were concerned was that this represented a deterioration in the quality of the diet. With the exception of milk and vegetables, the amount of 'protective foods' in the diet had markedly decreased (Fig. 5.1).[2] But the predicted health consequences of such a change in dietary pattern were not fulfilled. Far from deteriorating, the health of the nation appeared, if anything, to improve. The maternal, infantile and neonatal death rates fell steadily to the lowest ever recorded.[3] The average height and weight of schoolchildren increased by 1.5 and 6.7 per cent respectively. And a Ministry of Health nutritional survey of 20,235 children after six years of war and rationing could find only nine with evidence of frank nutritional deficiency disease.[1]

This epoch of improvement in the basic indices of the nation's health would have been remarkable in peacetime, let alone under the duress of war, and is certainly difficult to explain. Several factors may have contributed. Rationing had the effect of redistributing food towards the least well-off, annulling the gross inequalities of the pre-war years. Mothers and children in particular benefited from an increase in certain foods, and the growth of antenatal

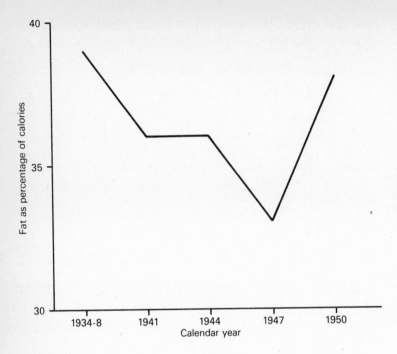

Fig.5.1 *The proportion of fat in the British diet (as a percentage of total calories) fell markedly during the war years*

services during these years brought many women into contact with preventive health services early in their pregnancies, which may have influenced the maternal and infant mortality rates. It is probable, furthermore, that the evacuation of children out of the cities in the early years of the war allowed them to grow up in an altogether healthier environment. But there is still some uncertainty as to whether the nutritional changes of the war years contributed to the better health of the nation. The trends noted in mortality statistics and the vital measurements of children were, after all, only a continuation of what had been taking place since the turn of the century.

For the moment, though, it is enough to observe that a decline in the absolute amount of 'protective' foods in the national diet, especially meat and dairy foods – a major change in the pattern of nutrition opposite to that advocated by Boyd Orr and the expert committees of the 1930s – had not resulted in a major deterioration in health. The scientific thesis that major increases in consumption of these foods were necessary to improve health had been critically tested by a natural experiment and found to be in error. Rather the results suggested that as long as people had sufficient calories and a moderately balanced diet, it did not really matter what that diet was.

Given this, it is also interesting to enquire whether that other truism of the 1930s – the nutritional superiority of brown compared to white bread – was equally valid. This is exactly what two British nutritionists, R. A. McCance and Elsie Widdowson, set out to discover at the end of the war.[4,5] Once again, as with Henrietta Chick's experiments on rickets in Vienna in the 1920s, the plight of children in a post-war world was the setting of the experiment.

In 1947, under the auspices of the Medical Research Council, McCance and Widdowson travelled to Wuppertal, an industrial town in the Ruhr valley made wealthy by the presence of the vast German pharmaceutical company IG Farbenindustrie. It had been bombed heavily with incendiary and high-explosive devices on several occasions from 1943 onwards, causing homelessness and deprivation on a massive scale. It was here that the nutritionists found two orphanages in which to conduct their famous experiment: 'On the nutritive value of bread and on the effect of variation in the extraction rate of flour on the growth of the undernourished.'

The orphanages contained 320 children in all, aged from 4 to 15. Food was at a premium as rationing applied to all ages. Breakfast was bread, jam and ersatz coffee; lunch was vegetables or vegetable soup. In the evening it was bread with a little butter, sausage, fish or cheese. One ounce of cooked meat was eaten on Sunday and there was half a pint of milk a week. Compared to the average diet of pre-war British schoolchildren, these German orphans were eating one-tenth as much meat, one-quarter as much milk and half as much butter and margarine, the deficit in calories being made up with almost indigestible amounts of potatoes, vegetables and bread, the last comprising more than 70 per cent of their calorie intake.

Despite this spartan diet the children appeared lively and energetic, but were small for their age. The heads of the orphanages did a deal with the British nutritionists, agreeing to comply with the proposed experiment in exchange for further limitless supplies of calories in the form of different types of bread. It was relatively straightforward to divide the children into groups and by giving them, in addition to their standard diet, breads of different degrees of refinement, test the critical question as to whether brown bread really was nutritionally superior to white. Seven types of bread were used, ranging from refined white to completely unrefined brown, one lot being further fortified with vitamins and iron.

The results at the end of the year were amazing in their consistency (Fig. 5.2). Irrespective of whether they were eating white or brown bread, fortified or unfortified, the children in each group put on exactly the same amount of weight and height and had impressively caught up with the normal measurements for children of their age: 'One of the most striking findings in the investigation and perhaps the most unexpected one, was the remarkable way in which the general condition of all the children improved.' Visitors to the orphanages who saw the children towards the end of the experiment 'all agreed they were in excellent physical shape. They were unable to pick out children as belonging to a particular bread group.'

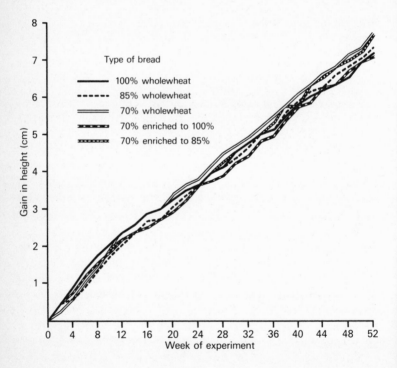

Fig.5.2 *The children in the Wuppertal experiment had the same rate of growth, irrespective of what type of bread they were given*

McCance and Widdowson concluded this part of their report:

> No difference could be found between the nutritional values of the breads, and since the children grew at a very satisfactory rate and no signs of deficiencies appeared it may be concluded that all the diets supplied the children with the nutrients known and unknown which they required.

So even in the exceptional circumstances where children had for several years been receiving a spartan diet sufficient to impede their growth, it seemed to make little difference whether they consumed refined bread from which the thiamin-containing husk had been removed or the nutritionally approved unrefined product. Again, as with the experience of the British diet in wartime, it appeared that the most important thing was to ensure sufficient calories within the context of a moderately balanced diet. The messianic claims for the unique virtues of unrefined bread as essential for the prevention of illness could not be sustained.

Reviewing their experience several years later, McCance and Widdowson made the following observations:

> The experiments showed firstly that wheat flour has a food value for growing children far beyond that usually allocated to it in recent years. The implications of this are great, particularly in parts of the world where flesh foods and milk are scarce and expensive. Secondly they made clear that unenriched white flour was just as valuable a constituent of the diets used at the orphanages as whole wheaten bread. Only under exceptional circumstances was it likely to fail – as in the absence of all vegetables and animal protein from the diet.[6]

Neither of these experiments, that of the wartime change in the national diet or the Wuppertal experience, seemed to have much influence on the nutritional beliefs that had been formulated in the 1930s. Success brings its own rewards and that of the wartime food policy in feeding the population at a time of national emergency obscured the fact that it had effectively disproved the experts' advocacy in the pre-war years of a major increase in dairy food and meat consumption. Neither did the Wuppertal experiment prompt a re-evaluation of the beliefs in the unique beneficial properties of brown bread. With the end of rationing, the public reverted to its traditional customs and the myths lived on.

If anything, indeed, belief in the importance of milk as therapeutic in building healthy bones increased, and was further reinforced in the post-war years by the growing stigmatisation of carbohydrate foods, especially bread and potatoes as being fattening. It was a belief that owed less to science than to powerful imagery (in this case an unhealthy, stodgy, potato-eating working class contrasted to a lean and tall dairy-eating upper class), since a given amount of dairy foods contains more calories than its equivalent in carbo- hydrate foods, and can therefore truly be said to be more fattening.

But that leaves unanswered one very important question. If the pre-war thesis of the need for a markedly increased consumption of meat and dairy foods had not been confirmed by experiment, because the nation's health had improved even though protective food consumption declined, these must mean there was something wrong with the evidence that had been used to suggest the contrary.

Boyd Orr's study *Food, Health and Income* had determined the extent of malnourishment by showing that half the population were failing to fulfil their Recommended Daily Allowances for certain nutrients. He had, in addition, used the differential in height between schoolboys from the two ends of the class spectrum as evidence of chronic malnourishment, without demonstrating that children from the lower social classes were genuinely malnourished. So two questions arose. Did the RDAs have any meaning; and was the height differential reflected in a health differential?

The answers to both these questions are to be found in a survey, *Family, Diet and Health*,[7] conducted in 1937 only one year after Boyd Orr's much more famous study. It replicated almost exactly Boyd Orr's findings, confirming the wide differential in food con- sumption patterns between the social classes, but went one step further by attempting to see whether the different pattern of food intake between the classes was reflected directly in measurements of physique and health.

Consider first the RDAs. The discovery that a deficiency of a vitamin or mineral in the diet led to conditions such as beriberi and rickets encouraged scientists to try to define how much and what people should be eating across the whole spectrum of food. This was done by taking a given nutrient such as calcium and assessing experimentally on animals how low its intake had to fall before a recognised deficiency state appeared. The results were then ex- trapolated to humans, adding a wide safety margin to take into account the range of requirements between individuals and addi- tional amounts that might be needed in case of illness. On this basis the person drawing up the RDA then decided on a figure.

This appears quite straightforward but the application of this knowledge when conducting nutritional surveys is fraught with problems. First it is necessary to find out what people have been eating: can the interviewee recall what he had for dinner last Saturday, and how much? There is already considerable scope for imprecision here. Then the scientist has to convert what was eaten into amounts of specific nutrients (how much iron in a slice of beef?) by referring to Food Composition Tables, the value of which is uncertain even to nutritionists.

> There are two schools of thought about Food Composition Tables. One tends to regard the figures as having the accuracy of atomic weight determinations. The other dismisses them as valueless on the grounds that a foodstuff may be so modified by the soil, the season or the rate of growth that no figure can be a reliable guide to its composition.[8]

Even when a figure is arrived at – for instance that last week a particular person consumed 4 grams of calcium – a whole new area of imprecision arises: how can one be sure that this is an adequate amount for one person compared to another? There is enormous variation in individual food requirements. A lumberjack will obviously need more than a sedentary secretary, but there are individuals of the same age, sex and occupation who consistently eat twice as much as their peers; some infants eat more than eighteen-year-old adolescents; some individuals can maintain a steady body weight on 1,500 calories per day, others need twice that figure.

The intentions of those drawing up the RDAs may be well-meaning but the application of their figures to the real world is by definition almost impossible. Uncertainty about what people eat, what is in the food they eat, and what an individual's requirement may be, makes most deductions hypothetical. The lack of precision is shown by the variability in the national RDAs of fifteen Western European countries.[9] From one to another country the protein requirement varies twofold from 60 to 120 grams; for calcium threefold; for vitamin A threefold from 30 to 100 mg. Someone living in Germany and consuming 300 mg of calcium per day is fulfilling his dietary norms, while in Britain he would be designated calcium deficient. By moving these figures up or down, millions of people can at a stroke change from being 'malnourished' to being 'overnourished'. So did Boyd Orr's specified RDA goals of optimal nutrition have any basis in biological fact?

Calorie intake provides an obvious test. Too few and one goes hungry and loses weight, too many and one is overeating and likely to become obese. According to the 1937 survey *Family, Diet and*

Health, only those in income group 3 were consuming the right amount of calories according to the Recommended Daily Allowances. Those above ate too many, those below too few. The citizens from Bow and Bethnal Green in the lowest income class (group 1), had only 60 per cent of the required calorie intake: 'Yet the clinical data did not show the children of these families to be semi-starved.' At the other end of the scale, those in income group 6 were deemed to be consuming a large excess of calories, and again there was no evidence to suggest that children from these families were overfed. The same was true of mineral and vitamin intake. Specific postulated deficits in calcium did not show up as evidence of bone deformities, or of vitamin A (important for vision) with evidence of visual defects.

Indeed in the whole of the survey there was not one example where the failure to achieve an RDA of any given nutrient was reflected in biological functioning. RDAs were meaningless as indicators of whether any section of the population was chronically malnourished or not, and their use as evidence that half the population were thus afflicted had no basis in reality. Boyd Orr's carefully constructed scientific case, indicting the diet of large sections of the population, was based on a pseudoscientific set of apparently arbitrary figures.

Nevertheless, it might still have been possible that the height differential he observed between social classes was reflected in a health differential. So how many children actually were malnourished – that is, had clinical evidence of nutritional deficiency disease and might therefore have benefited from major improvements in their diet?

The Ministry of Health kept its own statistics on malnutrition based on the annual examination of schoolchildren. These figures showed that before the First World War malnutrition indeed affected up to 20 per cent of children, but that there had been a steady improvement and that for the period 1929–32 'malnutrition requiring treatment' affected only 1 per cent.[10] There was a misleading element in these overall statistics, as they might have concealed areas in which the figure was 20 or 30 per cent. There certainly were great anomalies in the figures as presented: comparable areas in Northumberland, for instance, would return rates of between 0.5 and 7.5 per cent. Malnutrition appeared prevalent in some small cathedral towns, but virtually non-existent in some impoverished areas. Nonetheless, Sir Robert McCarrison had made claims in his prestigious public lectures in 1936 – claims that had been taken seriously by the Opposition in the recurrent debates on malnutrition in the House of Commons – that the real rate of malnutrition was several times that of the official figures. Who was right?

Here again *Family, Diet and Health* is useful as it specifically looked for evidence of malnutrition in children. The examination took three forms: physical measurements of height and weight; blood tests to detect anaemia (anaemia can be an indicator of poor nutrition if there is insufficient iron in the diet); and the diagnosis of clinical conditions caused by poor nutrition such as rickets, related ailments like knock knee, flatfoot and skeletal deformities; skin and eye infections, inflammation around the gums and mouth (associated with deficiencies of the vitamin B group) and catarrh and bronchitis.

The height and weight measurements showed a steady rise from the lowest income section (group 1) to the highest (group 6). The blood test for anaemia showed no difference between the classes: 'It seems safe to conclude that the haemoglobin levels do not change significantly with changing economic and nutritional circumstances', the survey observed. And the only clinical condition commoner among the lower social classes was bronchitis: 'This was the only marked trend with food expenditure.' Rather naively, the report added: 'It is not known whether bronchitis has any significant relation to nutrition.' (Bronchitis is in fact caused by poor housing rather than poor nutrition.)

By any criteria this was a damning result. A whole edifice of nutritional wisdom concerning widespread malnourishment and illness due to an impoverished diet seemed to have no basis in reality. Rather, it appeared that irrespective of expenditure on food, children somehow managed to be resiliently healthy, or at least that ill health appeared evenly distributed across the classes. Perhaps not surprisingly, this study, which effectively disproved the claims of the nutritionists of the 1930s, was not released for public scrutiny until well after the war when the reputations of the scientists involved were unlikely to be damaged.

The failure to find objective evidence for the claims of the 1930s explains why the reduction in protective foods in the war years did not have a deleterious effect on health. If in the first place there was no problem arising out of insufficient protective foods, reducing the amounts of these foods in the nation's diet would not have resulted in deterioration of the nation's health. So it is necessary to seek explanations for the widespread nutritional beliefs of those times outside the strict realms of science. Some of these explanations have already been encountered and it is worth reviewing them briefly.

There was obviously a strong ideological and emotional appeal in the promotion of the virtue of dairy foods. The greater height of children from the upper social classes (albeit less significant than suggested) was considered socially and culturally desirable, and the message was reinforced by the simplistic but powerful imagery that presented dairy foods as replete with 'bone- and flesh-forming material' which uniquely contributed to growth.

Even more important was the medical context within which the beliefs were held. The potency of the discovery that vitamins played a role in health came just at the time when the 'germ' theory of disease, which for so long had dominated medical thinking, was becoming less productive in providing novel insights. The simple reason for this was that most of the important disease-causing bacteria had already been discovered. Yet it seemed that the explicative power of the germ theory might be mirrored in the discovery that the absence of vital ingredients in food caused illness. This led to the belief that humans behaved like automatons which could only function if all the right ingredients were taken in the right amount at the right time. Illness, in the form of dietary deficiency, was due to an absence or insufficiency of these ingredients and the medical challenge was to ensure that as many people as possible were in receipt of the right ingredients – that is, were obtaining the optimal diet. The importance of the discovery of the vitamins was not balanced by a universal appreciation of the complexity of the nutritional processes by which the body can resiliently accommodate very different dietary patterns.

Furthermore, it is significant that despite many important advances in the understanding of the nature of disease, the medical profession remained very short on specific remedies, and would remain so until the therapeutic revolution of the post-war years. As it is distressing to care for the sick without the means to cure them, the idea that a perfectly constituted diet might both prevent and be a specific remedy for disease was very attractive. The strength of nutrition in these times was a reflection both of the importance of its real discoveries, and of the absence of other explanations and cures for illness.

But probably most significant in the widespread appeal of the contemporary dietary wisdom was the political context within which the nutritional beliefs operated. The widespread poverty and unemployment of the 1930s engendered both a simple analysis – that they were caused by the 'internal contradictions of capitalism' – and speculative and utopian solutions ranging from reform to revolution. These were mirrored in nutrition, in the shape both of the false analysis that attributed much illness to diet and its utopian solution of optimum nutrition as 'a state of well being such that no improvement can be effected by diet'. At a time when radicalism was so logical a political position because of the gross inequalities in society, it is perhaps not surprising that inequalities in the distribution of food were seen as having a profounder significance than they really possessed.

Boyd Orr and other experts used the terminology of science, 'objective' criteria of dietary adequacy, and their credibility as dispassionate observers of the human condition to demonstrate apparently widespread hunger and gross deficiencies in diet. They thus found a ready audience in a political movement which used those observations to promote fundamental political changes in society. The moral issue is whether they were justified in exploiting, wittingly or unwittingly, the political prejudices of the day to promote their nutritional ideas. There could be no doubt that there was inequality, and it was nonsensical that good-quality foods were being poured away when at minimal cost to the state they could be distributed to those who might benefit from them. But did that legitimate the misuse of science?

They were, in a complex way, serving two incompatible masters. Serve science alone, and the only result of their studies was to confirm what was already and for ever known – that there were inequalities in food distribution between classes. But to serve the interests of the people as they perceived them meant proving, in terms that the public and politicians could understand, that there was an identifiable medical problem arising out of those inequalities which could only be resolved by the institution of their nutritional prescriptions.

There were some at the time who understood these issues. In 1936 Robert Hutchinson, Consultant Physician at the London Hospital, pointed out in the *British Medical Journal*:

The subject of nutrition may be regarded as the public health 'stunt' of the moment. Unfortunately it is a subject that has got badly mixed up with politics with the consequence that much of the writing about it is of a tendentious nature. What is the 'optimum level of nutrition'? Should we aim as some enthusiasts would have us do at feeding children in such a way as to produce the maximum growth and development of which each is capable? If we succeed in this are we sure we have benefited the child?[11]

The Professor of Physiology at Glasgow University returned to the theme the following year: '. . . as to the extent of "malnutrition" it has given rise in recent times to great debate much of it extraordinarily ill informed . . . these would-be experts darken counsel by words without knowledge.'[12]

It was, however, an ordinary physician, Dr Lindsay Batten, whose contemporary commonsensical observations in 1936 provided perhaps the best refutation of the grand visions of the 1930s:

> I surely cannot be alone in being perplexed by the present wave of enthusiasm for nutrition. Eminent men tell us over the wireless of a 'new science of nutrition', and in our own journals we are told that nutrition is by far the single most important factor in the preservation of health. I gather that what we eat, rather than where or how we live, what is our work, who were or are our parents or what infections we encounter determine our stature, physique, immunity, or liability to sickness and even our mental outlook. I also gather that this is a new discovery, but whose or on what evidence based I am not told. Sometimes it almost seems to have been revealed.
>
> I find it very difficult to accept the dominating importance of diet and this for two reasons. First I should never have guessed that the broad facts of history bore out this contention. I should have thought on the contrary, that man had proved able in different places and different epochs to live, thrive, work, do great deeds and think high thoughts on an astonishing diversity of diets.
>
> Secondly, it is my lot to practise chiefly among people who are well fed according to the best modern standards. In general these people are healthy. Their children usually grow taller than those of the poorer classes, their young men and women are good physical specimens though I doubt if they would show up really well besides fisher folk, farm labourers or navvies. They do not get scurvy or rickets.
>
> But I know of no disorder occurring among the common folk of London to which the well fed are immune. The acute specific fevers attack them, they are prone to infections of the upper air passages and tonsils, they are smitten suddenly by appendicitis, pyelitis, cholecystitis, fibrositis and neuritis. They get staphylococcal infections of the skin. They get cancer. Their childbearing is not always free from misadventure. Some grow old before their time. Many are prey to illfound fears and cannot be happy. In fact they are heir to all the common ills of the flesh. It is what a man

does, and when he does it and what constitution he has inherited that determines his state of health rather than what he eats. We do a poor service to the community by preaching the easy doctrine of effortless health through food.[13]

Perhaps these judgements are too harsh. Serious evidence of malnourishment and food-related illness may have been absent – but at least it instigated social measures which allowed many children to enjoy free school milk that would otherwise have been thrown away. The poorer social classes may not have been as unhealthy as was suggested, but the economic system which condemned so many to a dreary diet was difficult to condone. And it was not really the fault of the experts if their scientific pronouncements were taken up and exploited by ambitious politicians.

Nonetheless, 'bad science makes worse social policy'. Scientists can practise bad science in the privacy of their own laboratories and the world is unaffected. But when bad science becomes the basis of policies that will affect ordinary people's lives, it has a tendency to procure unexpected and undesirable consequences.

The nutritional beliefs of the 1930s had at least two such consequences. They vitiated for nearly thirty years attempts to provide solutions to the problem of world hunger; and the practice in the war years of supplementing the foods with extra vitamins to prevent nutritional diseases that were at least very rare led to a completely new and lethal disease in young children.

The founding of the Food and Agriculture Organization (FAO) at the end of the Second World War was, like all the international organisations spawned at that time, inspired by the idealist notion that the institutionalisation of co-operation between countries would prevent a repetition of the tensions that had led Europe into two World Wars in thirty years. Its first Director General was Sir John Boyd Orr who had spent the war years canvassing for a 'world food plan', based on an analysis remarkably similar to that which had uncovered 'widespread malnutrition' in Britain in the 1930s, except on a much grander scale:

The kind of diet which man requires for health has been well established . . . yet the diets consumed by the greater part of mankind are nutritionally unsatisfactory . . . leading to impaired physical development, ill health and untimely death . . . malnutrition is found in all classes and all nations . . . in the USA and Western Europe affecting between 20 to 30 per cent of the population. . . . The diets of the great mass of the population in the East are grossly deficient in terms of any standard of adequacy . . . some 75 per cent of the 1,650 million inhabitants of Asia have a diet far below the standard for health.[14]

Such a drastic situation required drastic remedies, and in 1946 Boyd Orr proposed that a World Food Board be set up under the auspices of the FAO.

The Board would provide on request by any food-deficient country long-term loans to enable it to purchase surplus foods from food-exporting countries . . . the loan was to be free of interest or repayment of capital until hunger and abysmal poverty had been eliminated. . . . (The Board) would have authority to buy and hold stocks in countries with an exportable surplus of storable foods not immediately marketable.[15]

The principle was simple and humane; those with were to give to those without, but the proposals entailed not only the provision of substantial sums of money but also the handing over to international control of important national functions which governments naturally regarded as vital to the management of their own economies.

Boyd Orr's proposals failed, vetoed by the countries of the Western alliance and he retired a few months later, was ennobled, received the Nobel Prize for Peace and devoted himself to the cause of world government. But the perspective that delineated the scope of the problem of 'world hunger' lived on in the philosophy of the FAO. Boyd Orr had said that 'a lifetime of malnutrition and actual hunger is the lot of at least two-thirds of mankind', and over the following years, the FAO propagated this myth – there were variously 500 million, 750 million or 1,000 million undernourished in the world, calculations based on designating whole countries as being underfed because their figures of agricultural production did not achieve an arbitrary figure of required 'calories per head of population'. The calculations were not specific measures of malnourishment but of the relative poverty of the underdeveloped world: a problem of such political and social complexity as apparently to deny solution.

The problem for institutions such as the FAO, however, is that to justify their existence they have to come up with solutions. And so arose the concept of the 'protein gap' or 'protein crisis', later to become the 'protein fiasco'. As Boyd Orr had discovered malnourishment on a large scale in Britain between the wars due to insufficient consumption of dairy foods, the international agencies in the 1950s decreed that the problem of world hunger was caused not simply by people having insufficient to eat but rather by their having insufficient protein in their diets. The solution therefore required a major increase in production and consumption of protein.

The germ of this idea came from the description of a particular type of childhood malnutrition called kwashiorkor. The vast majority (about 95 per cent) of the starving children in the world suffer from a condition known as marasmus, caused by a dreary set of events. The victims will usually have been weaned early and abruptly, and then fed with dilute milk in unhygienic conditions. This in turn leads to repeated infections, particularly of the gut. The consequent diarrhoea is inadequately treated with fluid and calorie replacement. By now the children are the skin and bone tragedies so well known to the Western world from its television screens.[16]

Kwashiorkor is a different illness and confined almost exclusively to sub-Saharan Africa. These children are breast-fed for protracted periods of a year or more and gradually weaned on to the starchy foods so prevalent in those areas which are rich in carbohydrate but contain no good-quality protein. Acute infections follow and the child develops the features of kwashiorkor – swollen limbs, ulcerated skin, apathy and muscle weakness.

The difference between these two distinct clinical pictures of malnutrition is believed to be the poor quality and deficient protein in the diet of the children of sub-Saharan Africa. But regardless of the fact that kwashiorkor is a form of malnourishment affecting only a small percentage of the world's starving children, this protein deficit was seized on by the international agencies and became the explanation for *all* malnutrition; 'the most serious and widespread nutritional disorder known to medical and nutritional science'. As one of the leading protagonists argued:

> Much more than deficiency in calories it is deficiency in protein that threatens the development of the human race. . . . It is difficult to arrive at a precise estimate of the protein gap but it is certain that the deficit is so great that all the provisional objectives of production of protein foods for the next decades have no chance under any circumstances of being fulfilled.[17]

Now if there was a protein 'gap', as this hypothetical deficiency in the world supply of protein was described, that meant it had to be filled: 'The number-one problem for the Food and Agriculture

Organization and for national agricultural departments is the production of protein foods of good quality.' But what to fill it with?
And so arose the idea that in a world replete with natural sources of
food, the problems of the starving millions could only be solved by
manufacturing artificial protein foods. This task became the main
practical thrust of the activities of the food agencies from 1950 to
1971.

The results were disastrous, as a contemporary nutritionist
describes:

> Scores of these food mixtures have been produced but the
> majority have never reached commercial production and most of
> the others sooner or later proved financial failures. Today 'In-
> caparina', the most publicised mixture, costs nearly four times as
> much as the cornmeal it replaces and would use up more than
> one-sixth of a Central American peasant's daily wage to feed
> a twelve-month-old child . . . elsewhere another product sells
> mainly as pet food. There is not a single study to show that these
> mixtures can justify under practical field conditions the extrava-
> gant claims made for them.[18]

Fish protein concentrate provided the most spectacular example
of this farcical enterprise:

> Over a period of thirty years technologists were set the task of
> extracting protein from fish, they freed it from fat, deodorised it
> and with considerable difficulty ground it into an impalpable
> powder. . . . impoverished communities supplied with the con-
> centrate then declined to eat it. The final twist in this strange
> episode in the history of applied science which ultimately broke
> the spirit of those who had engaged themselves in the project and
> spent 20 million dollars came when the Food and Drugs Adminis-
> tration denied them the right to distribute the product on the
> grounds that, containing as it did the heads, tails, bones and
> scales and worst of all the intestines of the fish it contravened the
> health regulations as specified in the so-called 'filth test'. For
> twelve years the adamant authority held out. By the time they
> relented the myth was pricked and the project allowed quietly to
> crumble away.[19]

The myth-pricking came in 1975 when two scientists delivered the
coup de grâce in a classic paper which showed that while some
people undoubtedly have too little to eat, there are virtually no
circumstances in which communities are likely to suffer from a
specific protein deficit.[20] As the physiologist Starling had observed

years earlier: 'look after the calories and the protein will look after itself'. Indeed, only in the exceptional situation of the vulnerable children of sub-Saharan Africa will poor-quality protein cause a specific illness.

It seems incredible that for twenty years a vast international organisation such as the FAO should have endorsed such a simple-minded analysis and absurd solution to the problem of world hunger, but it did. The cost in time and money of all the research and development projects, of the numberless meetings of experts and concerned politicians, is at least finite. The cost to all the children lost in the scourge of malnutrition whose lives might have been saved were it not for this massive wastage of human and financial resources is incalculable. The source and inspiration for all this wasted activity is fully located in the inaccurate predictions and messianic hopes of the World Food Board.

Today wiser counsels prevail. The protein gap, the 'number-one nutritional priority', has ceased to exist. The numbing and meaningless estimates of the numbers of the world hungry are less frequently heard. The answers to the problem of feeding the world seem to lie where they always have done – not in the reports of nutritional experts but in the prospects of economic progress and political stability. The cataclysmic predictions of the post-war years have been muted by the obvious success of the vast continent of Asia in feeding itself.

The second unanticipated and deadly consequence of the nutritional certainties of the 1930s arose from the uncritical enthusiasm for vitamins. Not only was brown bread much superior to white because it retained the all-important thiamin, but foods could only benefit from having vitamins added to them; and vitamins in their pure form were promoted as essential for the maintenance of health. This enthusiasm was enormously strengthened during the Second World War, as Magnus Pyke recalls from his years working at the Ministry of Food:

> Because calculations implying that the food supply available to the fifty-odd million population of embattled Britain would provide insufficient calcium, chalk was added to bread to remedy the situation. Estimates suggested that the total thiamin concentration of the nation's food provided less than the tables of requirements laid down so synthetic thiamin was added to the bread.

High among the nutritional deficiency diseases that the planners hoped to prevent by vitamin supplementation was rickets. Accordingly, dried milk was fortified with vitamin D, as were babies' rusks and cereals, and a bonus of vitamin D-rich cod-liver oil was widely available through child welfare clinics. When it came to vitamins one could not have too much of a good thing – an idea exploited by commercial suppliers who further enriched the nation's vitamin D supply with proprietary preparations.

In the early 1950s doctors in Britain started to notice that some children were being born with similar and bizarre facial features, most notably a peaking of the ears. They were rapidly dubbed 'elfin children' and found to be deaf and mentally retarded. Another group of children, although apparently normal at birth, failed to put on weight, were anorexic, suffered from recurrent vomiting and constipation, and eventually died.[21] The common feature linking these two groups was a markedly elevated level of calcium in the blood, and it soon became apparent that this was because they or their mothers had been receiving excessive supplements of the vitamin that facilitates the absorption of calcium from the gut and its uptake by bone, the vitamin that prevents rickets – vitamin D.

However, vitamin D differs from other vitamins in that it is also manufactured in the skin under the influence of sunlight, while the amount in the diet (usually of the order of a few micrograms per day) is usually a relatively insignificant source. Examining the vitamin D intake of the children with the elevated levels of calcium in the blood soon showed that they or their mothers had been receiving ten to forty times the amount usually obtained from food; and these toxic levels of the vitamin were leading to very high calcium levels in susceptible children with lethal consequences. The inappropriate intervention of nutritional science had created a novel disease – idiopathic hypercalcaemia of infancy.

As the number of cases escalated, with up to 100 a year in the early 1950s, it became imperative rapidly to curtail the liberality with which vitamin D was being dispensed. Clinics cut back on their free provision, commercial companies were encouraged to remove their products from the market and with this done there was a welcome decline in the incidence of syndrome. A special investigation was set up by the British Paediatric Association, which compiled a report pointing out:

> The need for a dietary source of vitamin D is not well established. . . . Vitamin D appears to be obtained mainly from the

action of sunlight . . . what is known of the physiology of the vitamin suggests the body is better adapted to handling the vitamin from this source. The majority of the general population appear to have no need for any extra, and some individuals who habitually drink large quantities of milk would have intakes considerably in excess of requirements.[22]

The report considered the circumstances in which supplementing the diet with vitamin D might be of benefit, and concluded that it was necessary only for children who were vulnerable to rickets, particularly children of Asian origin whose darkened skin is less responsive to producing vitamin D from the diminished sunlight found in Britain.

The episode illustrates well a recurring problem in nutrition. It may be that certain 'at risk' groups will benefit from dietary changes or supplementation; but nutrition has a tendency to go for mass solutions; to try to prevent rickets, for instance, by giving *everyone* extra vitamin D. However, the observation that vitamins can be toxic when given in immoderate doses spelt the end of the mass solution principle, and encouraged instead a shift of policy towards focusing nutritional intervention on those who might need it. This sensible and commonsensical policy lasted for some fifteen years; but by the 1980s the lesson appeared to have been forgotten as once again nutrition expanded its ambitions and sought to change the diet of the whole nation. The pretensions of the new nutritional wisdom, as we shall see, were as ill-founded as those of the old, and its consequences potentially equally unfortunate.

There are two aspects to the history of nutrition in the early part of the present century. The first is the dedication and scientific rigour of those who set out to clarify and classify the composition of foods and the role of vitamins and minerals in human physiology. Their findings, although not perhaps of enormous practical significance to the Western world, were to prove of great benefit to those countries less privileged. The tenacity with which these scientists sought to unravel the secrets of this small but important aspect of human physiology is a tribute to the human spirit.

The second aspect could be called 'the search for relevance': the desire of doctors and scientists to find in these discoveries some universal solution for the ills of mankind. This required habits antithetical to the virtues that had made those discoveries possible: a tendentious overinterpretation and false extrapolation from the evidence, a lack of scientific rigour and common sense. It meant entangling the science of nutrition in politics and generated some resilient myths about the value of dairy foods and meat in the national diet. In certain instances its messianic solutions were positively harmful.

Exactly the same confusions are at work in the nutritional orthodoxies of the present day. Its wisdoms are the reversal of the old beliefs – meat and dairy foods are now 'saturated fats', stigmatised as the cause of the West's 'killer diseases' such as heart disease and cancer. But its claims to truth are no more founded in scientific fact or experiment than the myths it has superseded.

6
The Healthy Diet of 1980

We now move fast forward to the affectionately named 'swinging sixties'. The 1930s appear as a bad nightmare when, for a while, Western civilisation faltered, threatened from within by the consequences of economic stagnation, and from without by the hostile ideologies of Fascism and Marxism. But the system had proved itself remarkably resilient; the growth of the post-war economy had brought full employment and a rising standard of living for all classes.

The American Professor of Economics, J. K. Galbraith caught the mood and put a name to it: 'The Affluent Society'.

> The experience of nations with well being is exceedingly brief. Nearly all throughout history have been poor. The exception, almost insignificant in the whole span of human existence, has been the last few generations in the comparatively small corner of the world populated by Europeans. Here, and especially in the United States, there has been great and unprecedented affluence, which until now has been the accepted future.[1]

Farewell, Harry Pollitt: 'The stark reality is of a hungry Britain, badly fed, clothed and housed'. Now the reality was of a Britain that 'had never had it so good'. The new reality would bring with it a new nutritional wisdom.

It was not just the democratisation of affluence that distinguished the Western world from earlier epochs. For the first time in recorded history most of its citizens were living long enough to appreciate their good fortune – almost unnoticed, most people were now living out their biological lifespan. In 1911, the average citizen died thirty-eight years before his time, i.e. before his biological life expectancy; in 1950 this had fallen to seventeen years, and by 1980 to twelve years.[2] The problem of premature death had been almost completely eliminated. Death itself had not been defeated, no one had found the secret of immortality, but the pattern of disease had so altered that now the major causes of death were intrinsically related to the process of ageing and to the consequences of prolonging the lifespan. None of this is to suggest that the problem of disease had been solved – far from it. People remained vulnerable to a whole host of chronic non-fatal illnesses of uncertain cause such as diabetes, rheumatoid arthritis and multiple sclerosis, which medicine could alleviate but could not cure.

Three factors explain the difference over these eighty years. Firstly, there has been an enormous improvement in the prospects for survival of the very young (that is a marked fall in the perinatal mortality rate). Secondly, infectious diseases (especially tuberculosis) have been virtually eliminated as an important cause of death. Thirdly, everyone is just living longer.

Whereas in 1931 infectious diseases and tuberculosis accounted for as many as one-quarter of all deaths, by 1976 they had shrunk into insignificance and cancer and the circulatory disorders massively dominated the mortality statistics.[3,4]

If most people have a lifespan approximating to their natural life expectancy, it might be expected that the diseases they mostly do die of – circulatory disorders and cancer – would themselves be intimately related to the process of ageing. This is indeed the case. Examination of the incidence of these conditions by age shows that they are relatively rare until middle life, after which they escalate incrementally in succeeding decades. Far and away the most powerful predictor of these diseases is age, and indeed 75 per cent of deaths from both circulatory disorders and cancer occur in people over the age of 70 (Fig. 6.1).[5] By comparison, the incidence of non-age-related diseases like asthma remains fairly constant throughout life.

Why should life end with one or other of these categories of illness? Both arise from a failure of a dynamic system in the body. The cells of the body are dynamically dividing and replicating all the time, and over the years this process of division can go awry, resulting in a cancerous growth. (Cancer can of course occur in young children as well, although here its biology is different.) Similarly, the blood hurtles through the circulatory system day in, day out for years and the conduits of the system – the arteries – like any physical structure get worn down by stress. The legal require-

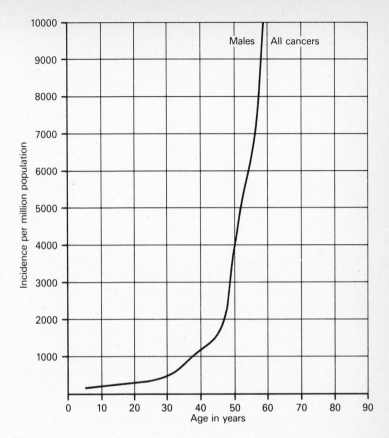

Fig.6.1 *The incidence of cancers rises dramatically with age, indicating that they are age determined*

ment to record a cause of death on the death certificate further swells the statistics as many who pass away quietly in their beds of 'old age' are deemed to have died from 'circulatory disorders'.

In order to push life expectancy to the ideal – that is, completely to eliminate the problem of premature death – it would be necessary to postpone these two categories of disease until as late as possible. But because they are largely related to age it will be impossible to eliminate the diseases themselves until the secret of immortality has been revealed (with the exception of those cancers where the cause is known, such as lung cancer – or where effective screening methods can catch them early, such as cervical cancer in the young).

No one has been able to provide a satisfactory explanation for the phenomenal improvements in life expectancy and health over the last eighty years. Medical progress has played a part but not nearly as significant as many imagine. Tuberculosis, for example, was in steep decline long before medicine discovered the drugs to deliver the *coup de grâce* to this once awesome 'captain of the armies of death'.[6] So we are reduced to generalisations: that improvements in housing and nutrition and lifestyles have strengthened our ability to resist infection, or reduced our exposure to infectious diseases; and that the same processes have also prolonged our lives. Anyone taking stock of the health of the nation in the 1960s might justifiably conclude that to live in the Western world was to live uniquely in a society where not only had relative prosperity become the norm, but where the elimination of premature and untimely death had all but been accomplished.

By the late 1970s, however, this vision of the extraordinary health of the Western world had been turned on its head. Its inhabitants were no longer the privileged beneficiaries of a society where most lived out their natural lifespan, but were rather besieged by an epidemic of killer diseases induced by affluence. These killer diseases, the circulatory disorders and cancers, were no longer the inescapable accompaniment of a long life, but 'diseases of civilisation'; and most prominent among their causes was the 'Western diet'.

By 1977 the Assistant Secretary of Health to the US Government was telling a Congress subcommittee:

> While scientists do not yet agree on the specific causal relationships, there is general agreement that the kinds and amounts of food we consume in our affluent society may be the major factor associated with the causes of cancer, circulatory disorders and other chronic illnesses.

The opinion was reinforced by Professor Mark Hegsted of Harvard School of Public Health: 'There is a great deal of evidence which strongly implicates, and in some instances proves, that the major causes of death and disability in the United States are related to the diet we eat.'[7]

Acting on this 'great deal of evidence', the committee under the chairmanship of Senator Edward McGovern produced in 1977 a report entitled 'Dietary Goals for the United States', which called for massive reductions in the consumption of meat and dairy produce as an important preventive measure against the epidemic. In 1983, in Britain, a report prepared by the National Advisory Committee on Nutrition Education (NACNE) came to the same conclusions, and popular nutritionists elaborated on its message: 'Leaders of the medical profession now have come to speak of a holocaust, which medicine can do nothing to check. Western food is the main single underlying cause of Western disease.'[8]

Human nutrition was once again a hot scientific and political issue, but its recommendations were now the exact opposite of those that had been proposed to eliminate the presumed widespread malnourishment of the 1930s. What had led to this change of heart?

In the changing pattern of disease this century, there have been two notable exceptions to the general trend in improvement in health. First, while the rates of most cancers have only increased at a level that reflects the growing longevity of the population, there has been an enormous increase in the number of deaths from lung cancer, which have risen fifty-fold in the last fifty years.[9] As we have seen, there is indisputable evidence to link this to a marked increase in cigarette smoking. Secondly, within the category of circulatory disorders, there has been a marked increase in early deaths from heart disease, especially among middle-aged men (Fig. 6.2).[10] In the decade prior to the McGovern and NACNE reports it had been argued with increasing conviction that just as the rise in lung cancer was due to smoking, so the rise in premature heart disease was due to the consumption of saturated fat – essentially dairy products and red meat. The wide acceptance of this 'diet-heart thesis' became the pillar which in turn sustained a much wider indictment of other types of food, especially salt and sugar, as important modifiable causes of many different diseases of the Western world: the diet-disease thesis. To understand how this nutritional edifice came into being, it is therefore first necessary to examine in more detail the most prominent of the 'diseases of civilisation' – heart disease.

There is no disputing the fact that from the 1920s onwards there was throughout the Western world a marked and inexorable increase year by year in early and unexpected deaths, predominantly among middle-aged men, attributed to 'heart disease'. By the 1950s it had become the commonest cause of premature death among males, afflicting one in five before the age of 65. It was a savage irony that as the countries of the West changed to place long life and prosperity within the reach of most, this phenomenon should arise to grab life away so suddenly and dramatically from so many before

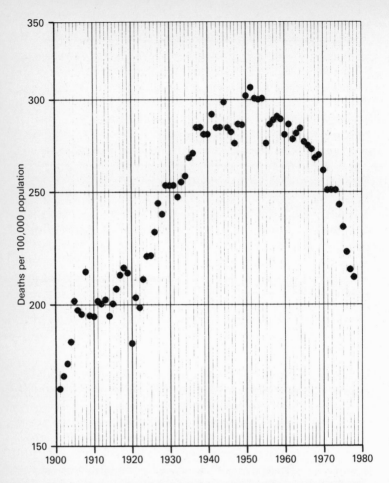

Fig.6.2 *Death rate from heart disease in the U.S. rose dramatically from 1920 to 1960 but has fallen as fast in the last two decades*

their time. This lethal and unpredictable disease, like AIDS in the mid-1980s, rapidly became a priority for medical research and its cause and prevention an obsession for the guardians of the public health.

The heart is a remarkable organ. The pump of life, it beats away 72 times a minute, 24 hours a day, 365 days a year for a lifetime, thrusting blood around the arteries, carrying oxygen, chemicals and the building bricks of cells to the furthest regions of the body. To perform this monumental task, the heart muscle itself must receive oxygen from three arteries called the coronary arteries. 'Heart disease', as commonly understood, is a disease of these arteries, and so is labelled coronary heart disease (CHD).

Most people develop in their arteries a condition known as atherosclerosis, which increases in severity over time. Its initiating mechanism remains obscure but early signs of the condition are known as 'atheromatous plaques' – patches of a porridge-like substance that accumulates in the lining of the arteries, consisting of a type of fat known as cholesterol and surrounded by fibrous tissue. These patches slowly increase in size and extent, narrowing the arteries and impeding the flow of blood. When they affect the coronary arteries, the blood flow to the heart muscle is similarly reduced, which can result in the four different and interconnected conditions of heart disease. The first is angina pectoris – literally a pain in the chest – first described by the distinguished eighteenth-century physician, Heberden:

> They who are afflicted with it are seized while they are walking (more especially if it be uphill, or soon after eating) with a powerful and most disagreeable sensation in the chest, which seems as if it would extinguish life if it were to increase or continue, but the moment they stand still, all this heaviness vanishes.

This is what happens. Imagine a man out for a walk. His pulse is beating away at 70 beats per minute and he feels fine. Then he comes to a small hill. This increases the amount of work his leg muscles have to perform and so the amount of oxygenated blood they need from the heart, and thus his pulse rate increases. But if the arteries to the heart are narrowed and the amount of blood passing through them is not sufficient to allow for the increased pulse rate, the heart muscle itself becomes relatively deprived of oxygen (or ischaemic). This is experienced as 'the most disagreeable sensation in the chest'. When the man stops and his pulse rate comes back down to normal, the heart muscle's need for extra oxygen declines and the pain goes away.

The second clinical condition is a 'heart attack' or coronary thrombosis (often shortened to a 'coronary'). Here a blood clot or 'thrombus' forms on top of an atheromatous plaque and the artery becomes completely blocked. The heart muscle beyond the blocked artery is absolutely deprived of oxygen and the patient experiences the same pain in the chest as angina pectoris but it lasts much longer. There are two consequences. Either the function of the heart muscle is so disrupted that it stops beating and the victim dies; or the damaged heart muscle beyond the blockage is repaired by fibrous tissue and the patient recovers.

The third condition is known as 'sudden death'. In this the victim – who may never have had any idea that he has heart disease – walks out one day and with no warning suddenly collapses and dies. For some reason and in a similar way to the acute event following a coronary thrombus, the heart muscle ceases to function properly. These cases of sudden death are recorded under the category of coronary thrombosis and are popularly understood to be heart attacks, but autopsy studies reveal that in less than one-third of cases is there actually evidence of a thrombus in the coronary arteries. In fact, the precipitating event leading to sudden death is not known.

Finally there is the category of 'chronic heart disease', in which, after recurrent heart attacks, so much of the heart muscle is replaced by fibrous tissue that it becomes incapable of pumping blood and 'fails'.

Because atherosclerosis is almost universal in Western societies, and because its severity increases with age, one would expect these four clinical conditions to have been around for a long time, at least among the elderly. But they have not and until the beginning of the twentieth century they were remarkably rare.[11] The greatest of all physicians at the turn of the century, William Osler, did not see a single case of angina till he had been in practice for twelve years. Coronary thrombosis or heart attacks were even rarer, being first described in 1912. The first paper in Britain to describe heart attacks was not published until 1925. It opens: 'In sudden thrombosis of the coronary arteries there may occur a very characteristic clinical syndrome which has attracted little attention in Britain and which receives scant attention in the textbooks.' The paper proceeds to describe three cases of an apparently new disease – coronary thrombosis.[12]

It is from 1925 that coronary thrombosis springs up from the mortality statistics to begin its relentless rise as an important, then *the* most important cause of death in middle-aged men. A condition first described in the British medical literature in 1925 would by 1950 be seen by a casualty officer in a busy hospital as many as three times in a single evening.

There are possible explanations for this apparent increase other than an absolute rise in incidence of the disease. The most obvious is that once a clinical syndrome is described, doctors diagnose it more often because now they can put a label on something they did not previously recognise. More importantly perhaps, a new disease changes the categories of causes of death recorded on death certificates – so deaths that might previously have been attributed to 'myocardial degeneration' now become 'coronary thrombosis', and the disease appears to be increasing much more rapidly than it really is. Nonetheless there is no doubt that coronary thrombosis grievously and exponentially increased in absolute incidence from the 1920s onwards. It is ultimately inconceivable that the specific clarity of the description of an attack with its 'life-extinguishing' heavy chest pain could have been missed or misinterpreted on a large scale by physicians of previous decades.

Sir Maurice Cassidy, Royal Physician, gave his opinions in the Harveian Oration of 1946:

> Curiously it was not until 1925 that McNee brought to the notice of physicians in this country the clinical picture of coronary thrombosis and the rapid increase in certification of death from coronary thrombosis must be partly attributable to this. Even so, I have the impression that coronary thrombosis is far more prevalent than it was. Looking through my notes of patients seen twenty or thirty years ago I come across occasional cases where I failed to recognise it, which now is the obvious diagnosis, but these cases are remarkably few.[13]

The significance of the historical development of heart disease is that it is so open to interpretation. If atherosclerosis is the underlying determining cause of the disease why were its apparent consequences – the clinical syndromes of angina, coronary thrombosis and sudden death – so rare before the twentieth century? And why, if it is a disorder that increases in severity with age, did it start to reap its grim harvest in middle age?

Put bluntly, it is the contention of the diet-heart thesis that the rise in heart disease over the last fifty years has been caused by the Western diet. In particular, consumption of dairy foods and meat is said to have raised the level of cholesterol in the blood and so increased the severity of atherosclerosis. It is worth looking at the evidence for this assertion in some detail, and especially at the links which connect cholesterol and heart disease.

Cholesterol is a 'lipidic compound' with numerous functions. It is an integral part of the architecture of the cell wall, as necessary to its stability as mortar in a brick wall. It is also transformed into a whole series of hormones, especially the sex hormones (testosterone in the male, oestrogen and progesterone in the female) and the steroid hormones involved in the control of inflammation.[14] As new cells are constantly being formed and the body requires a constant level of the sex and steroid hormones, there has to be a constant level of cholesterol circulating in the blood. So the first questions are: what controls the amount of cholesterol in the blood? Where does it come from and where does it go?

There are two sources of cholesterol. Some comes from food, for example eggs and avocados, but most (about four times as much) is made by the body itself in the liver. On the other side of the equation, cholesterol is continually being removed from the blood to be incorporated into the cell walls or form the basis of hormones; or it is being excreted in the bile. The whole is, then, a continuous process in which cholesterol is absorbed from the gut or made in the liver, transported through the arteries, and then taken up into cells or excreted. This description suggests that it would be difficult to influence the level of cholesterol in the blood by changing the diet. Food is only a minor source of the substance and its concentration in the blood is, like all physiological mechanisms, under the control of complex self-regulatory processes that ensure its level remains stable. Reducing the amount in the diet makes the liver manufacture more; increasing the amount in the diet means only that more is excreted.

Nonetheless, it was shown in the 1950s that making major changes in the diet, and particularly altering the ratio of saturated fat (essentially meat and dairy products) to polyunsaturated fat (essentially fats of vegetable origin and fish) can change the level of blood cholesterol – although the results are unpredictable, with large variation from one individual to another.[15] However, the actual evidence that cholesterol is involved in the process of atherosclerosis and so heart disease does not come from showing that manipulation of the diet can increase the amount of cholesterol in the blood. Instead it comes from the experience of a small group of people in the population with a defect in a gene that controls the protein that carries cholesterol. These people have very raised levels of cholesterol (the medical word is hypercholesteraemia). They develop very severe atherosclerosis and die from heart disease early in life.[16,17]

Most victims of heart disease, however, have 'normal' levels of blood cholesterol. This needs a little clarification. Measurement of any biological parameter in the body, be it height or weight or blood pressure or cholesterol in the blood, provides what is known as a 'bell' distribution, because the values obtained, when displayed graphically, resemble a bell (Fig. 6.3).[14] Most people lie around the average (i.e. the top of the bell), and decreasing numbers fall either below or above (i.e. make up the sides of the bell). Very few will have very low levels, very few will have very high levels. In the case of cholesterol, the majority at the top of the bell will have a level in the blood of around 220 mg in 100 mls (expressed as 220 mg per cent), but some (those with hypercholesteraemia) will have very high levels over 300 mg per cent. These will have a high rate of heart disease, but because they are relatively few in number compared to the majority with normal cholesterols, most cases of heart disease will be found in those with normal cholesterols. The important question therefore is whether it is possible to extrapolate from the experience of those few people with very high cholesterols to say anything valid about the experience of normal people. In other words, is cholesterol an important cause of heart disease for all, even those with normal levels; or is it merely an additive cause of heart disease in those with very high levels?

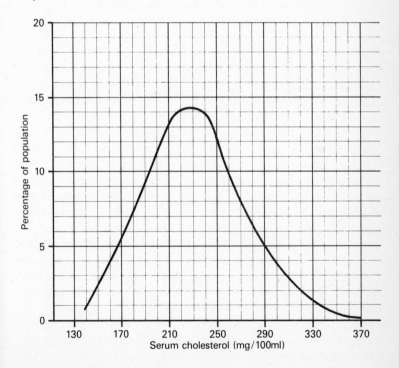

Fig.6.3 *Bell graph of the levels of blood cholesterol in the U.S. population*

Setting this question aside for the moment, it is now possible to see how the diet-heart hypothesis takes shape. The underlying cause of heart disease is presumed to be atherosclerosis, of which cholesterol is an important constituent. The evidence from those with high cholesterols due to a defect in the transport of this substance in the blood shows cholesterol to be important in at least some cases of the disease. Dietary manipulation studies show that it is possible to influence the level of cholesterol in the blood by changing the ratio of different types of fat consumed. Therefore the hypothesis argues that animal fat in the diet raises the cholesterol in the blood, which infiltrates the arteries, so increasing the severity of the atherosclerosis, which narrows the arteries to the heart, so causing heart disease. Accordingly, the massive rise in heart disease over the last fifty years should be explicable in terms of major changes in diet that particularly affect middle-aged men. Likewise, the remedy could be equally massive social intervention in order to change the national diet.

Important as this interpretation of events might prove to be, the immediate priority in the period just after the Second World War was seen to be the need to do something practical to influence the toll of the disease. And there seemed to be an answer at hand. It will be recalled that while the underlying cause of narrowing of the arteries might be atherosclerosis, the acute event in a heart attack is the clotting of the blood which forms a thrombus and occludes the coronary artery completely, resulting in the death of the heart muscle beyond. In 1939 a novel type of drug was discovered which -inhibited this process of clotting: the anticoagulant warfarin. It had an initial and very successful role as a rat poison, killing by inducing an internal haemorrhage. Perhaps it could be used to control the epidemic of heart disease? A patient who survived a heart attack was likely to have another one which could prove fatal, so why not give him the rat poison, reduce the blood's ability to clot and so prevent a further episode of thrombosis? What had proved lethal to rats could prove life-saving in man.

But did it work? Theoretically it should, but the only way to be sure was by conducting a therapeutic trial: give one lot of patients the drug, another a placebo, and sit back and watch what happened. The early trials were encouraging, but in the mid-1950s the pendulum gradually swung the other way. A typical study from Denmark concluded in 1962:

On the basis of our own results and those of others it cannot be ruled out that the use of anticoagulants in patients who have survived a heart attack exerts a certain prophylactic (protective) effect, but its effect on the course of the disease as manifested by mortality (i.e. the number who die from it) is very slight or nil.[18]

The largest of all trials organised by the Medical Research Council delivered the *coup de grâce* two years later: the difference in mortality rates between those on the anticoagulant and those on the placebo was negligible.[19]

Optimism turned to despair. Enormous energy had gone into trying to influence this fearful disease by a method which on theoretical grounds should have worked – but the outcome was a lemon. 'By 1970 everyone was weary, and felt alternative approaches must give more rewarding dividends . . . the coronary thrombosis (heart attack)–anticoagulant concept was abandoned by most through apathy.'[20]

These attempts to influence the disease might have been abandoned, but that did not mean the disease would go away. Medicine abhors a therapeutic vacuum, so if inhibiting the blood from clotting did not work an alternative had to be found. Emerging from the shadows with no serious challengers to its eminence, the diet-heart thesis was to dominate thinking about the disease for the next two decades. Its attraction was that it went further than tackling the empirical question of how to prevent someone with heart disease having another heart attack. Much more excitingly, it argued that the disease could be prevented in the West by a change of diet. And there appeared to be plenty of circumstantial evidence.

7
The Sources of Evidence

By the late 1940s the relentless rise in heart disease as a cause of premature death in middle-aged men was crying out for an explanation. The problem was where to start and the obvious place was at home. Take a group of people, study their lives, what they eat, how much they smoke, how much exercise they take, find out whether they are happy or unhappy, how heavy they are and how tall. And write it all down. As the years pass, nature will complete the study. Some will develop heart disease – and then it is back to the analysis again. What distinguishes those who died from heart disease from those who did not? It is possible to identify from all the information that was collected at the beginning of the study certain clues as to its cause, 'risk factors' for the disease?

As we saw in Chapter 1, identifying a risk factor for a disease does not necessarily mean identifying its cause. It might merely be an association; it might be an additional but not determinant factor in the disease in the same way that smoking is a risk factor for death from the pneumonia Legionnaire's disease. But a risk factor can be causal: smoking is both a risk factor for, and a cause of, lung cancer.

There have been many studies looking for the risk factors in heart disease, the most famous of which involved the citizens of Framingham, a small suburb of Boston, Massachusetts.[1] The Framingham study was started immediately after the Second World War and continues to the present day, and it has demonstrated certain powerful risk factors for the disease, particularly sex and age. It established that heart disease occurred predominantly in males and increased in incidence with age. (Another study from Britain identified social class as a further risk factor of this type, in that the disease was commoner among the lower than the upper social classes.)[2] Interesting as these risk factors might be, they are obviously of little value in treating or preventing the disease – it is not possible to change one's sex or age and only with difficulty one's social class. More important, then, was the discovery that other, modifiable characteristics of people's lives appeared to be risk factors: cigarette smoking, raised blood pressure (hypertension) and high levels of cholesterol in the blood (hypercholesteraemia). Furthermore, they had a compounding effect – the more risk factors, the higher the subsequent likelihood of a heart attack.

Equally important for the diet-heart thesis, however, were those things found not to be risk factors. In particular, the amount of fat in the diet of individuals neither predicted the level of cholesterol in the blood, nor the subsequent risk of heart disease.

The Framingham study thus provides no evidence in favour of the first link in the diet-heart thesis chain of causation – the link associating dietary fats with cholesterol levels in the blood; but it does provide evidence for the second link – those with high cholesterols had a higher risk of heart disease. Despite the fact that heart disease is frequently described as a 'lifestyle disease', the only aspect of lifestyle so far incriminated is smoking. To incriminate the main lifestyle factor – food, particularly animal fats – it is necessary to look elsewhere.

Given that there is a marked discrepancy in the incidence of heart disease between different countries, perhaps the answer is to be found here? In the early 1950s an American epidemiologist, Ancel Keys, conceived an ambitious plan to conduct a study like the one in Framingham, but involving seven countries. His 'Seven Country' study continues to be the linchpin of the diet-heart thesis.[3]

The countries chosen by Keys represented the extremes of incidence of the disease, from Japan – where it was very rare – to Finland, where it was untimely killing almost 50 per cent of the male population. In between were three Mediterranean countries – Greece, Yugoslavia and Italy – whose experience of the disease was similar to that of Japan; and the US and the Netherlands, whose experience was similar to that of Finland.

The Japanese contingent came from two small fishing villages. Their diet consisted of rice, soybean, vegetables in great variety, fish and other seafood. There was little fat in the diet and hardly any dairy produce. The Finns were also drawn from two small villages living in subarctic conditions; dairy produce and meat formed a major source of their calories. The Americans studied were a group of railway workers, as were the Italians. The Greeks from Crete and Corfu appeared to have a high fat intake but it was mostly in the form of the polyunsaturated fat, olive oil. The Yugoslav contingent consisted of a group of lecturers from the University of Belgrade.

The whole study was a masterpiece of logistic ingenuity. Eleven thousand men were weighed and measured, had their blood pressures and cholesterol levels recorded, and their smoking habits and dietary customs described. They then had to be followed up, their illnesses diagnosed and causes of death determined. Then, at five-yearly intervals, the results were analysed and written up. These showed that, in the countries studied, the amount of saturated fat (essentially animal fat) in the diet correlated both with the average level of cholesterol in each population and with the incidence of heart disease. The results are shown in the graph (Fig. 7.1): Japan appears in the bottom left-hand corner with low fat intake and low levels of heart disease, Finland in the top right-hand corner with high fat intakes and high levels of heart disease, and the other countries in between with their heart disease rates apparently related to their consumption of fat.

The next step in the development of the diet-heart thesis was to demonstrate that death rates from heart disease were in fact related to the presumed underlying cause – the extent of atherosclerosis

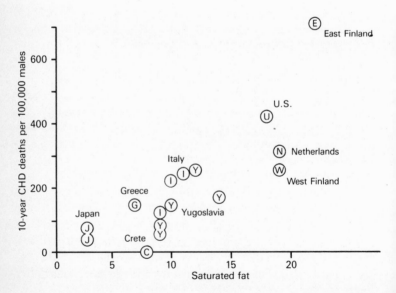

Fig.7.1 *The rate of heart disease in different countries is related to the amount of saturated fat (as a percentage of total calories) in the diet*

in the coronary arteries. This question was addressed in 1968 in another study of similar magnitude to that of Ancel Keys – The International Atherosclerosis Project.[4] This time 23,000 autopsy specimens from fourteen different countries were sent to one centre where pathologists busied themselves measuring the severity of atherosclerosis, the result being expressed as a percentage of the area of the coronary arteries with raised atherosclerotic plaques.

The results can be summarised as follows:

1. No society is free from atherosclerosis.

2. Within any society there is a wide scatter of severity of atherosclerosis for any given age group, ranging from nil to 100 per cent.

3. It is quite possible to have severe atherosclerosis even in societies with low fat intakes. Indeed the amount of fat consumed does not predict the severity of atherosclerosis. And

4. There are some people who die from heart attack with little or no atherosclerosis in the coronary arteries. Nonetheless,

5. If a comparison is made between countries, like the Seven Country study, death rates from heart disease appear to correlate with severity of atherosclerosis.

The next important piece of evidence in favour of the thesis came from studying what happens to migrants as they move from a society with a low fat intake and low rates of heart disease to one with a high fat intake and a high rate of heart disease. This has been done many times, but most importantly in the NI-HON-SAN study of 2,138 Japanese in Japan (NI), 8,006 Japanese in Honolulu (HON) and 1,842 Japanese in San Francisco (SAN). The results clearly demonstrate a rising incidence of heart disease as the Japanese migrants become progressively more Westernised – a change in incidence attributed to the increasing amount of fat in their diet.[5]

Two other pieces of evidence are frequently cited in favour of the thesis. If it is correct that the Western diet causes heart disease, then those in the West who do not eat a Western-style diet should have a lower incidence of the disease. The group most studied here has been the Seventh Day Adventists in the US, who as vegetarians have a low fat intake. They have 50 per cent less heart disease than the general population and, interestingly, much lower rates of cancer, respiratory disease and liver cirrhosis.[6]

Finally, there is the experience of the war years. During the German occupation, people in Western European countries suffered severe dietary restrictions compared to the US. And whereas the rate of deaths attributable to atherosclerosis in the US kept climbing during this period, they declined quite markedly in Scandinavian countries. Leaving aside problems of the validity of death certification at a time of war and the fact that the figures are all deaths attributed to 'atherosclerosis', rather than the 'premature deaths from heart disease' which the diet-heart thesis attempts to explain, these statistics are certainly impressive.[7]

And that is the scientific evidence in favour of the diet-heart thesis. The effort to implicate food in heart disease has certainly proved enormously expensive in terms of research, time and money. The studies described here are the most important and frequently cited, but they represent only a fraction of this vast exercise. Just adding together the 20,000 participants in the Framingham study, the 11,000 in the Seven Country study, the 12,000 in the NI-HON-SAN study and the 23,000 autopsies in the Atherosclerosis Project, gives a glimmering of the enormous scale of the enterprise.

Presented in this way, the evidence it has gathered appears convincing. The Framingham study shows heart disease to be a 'multifactorial disease' influenced by several different factors – age, sex, smoking, raised blood pressure and raised cholesterol levels. The evidence that animal fats can influence cholesterol levels and so cause the disease comes from comparing its incidence in different countries. The migrant studies suggest an environmental cause which could well be diet, because moving from one country and one dietary pattern to another influences an individual's risk of the disease. The low incidence of the disease among vegetarians and during the war years again suggests that food might be a vital factor.

But there are also gaps. Nobody has attempted to demonstrate that the phenomenal rise in heart disease in the Western world over the last five decades is actually related to increased fat consumption in the diet. And why, if animal fats cause heart disease, was the Framingham study unable to show a relationship between the amount of fat in the diet, the level of cholesterol and the subsequent risk of heart disease?

Similar gaps emerge when reviewing the evidence for the wider diet-disease thesis, which indicts the Western diet in a range of other killer diseases. Again the main source of evidence is the comparison of disease rates between countries and the effects of migration on the risk of disease; but again it is not possible to show within one country that those who suffer from these diseases consume more of the supposed dietary cause than those who do not. In fact, these gaps are immensely significant for both the diet-heart and the diet-disease theses. In order to understand their full import it is worth attending in a little more detail to three of the links most publicised by those who promote the latter: that between cancer and the Western diet; between 'fibre' and diseases of the gut; and between salt and the high blood-pressure which leads to strokes.

Diet and Cancer

In 1981, Sir Richard Doll and Richard Peto of Oxford University published a review of the relationship between diet and cancer.[8] This paper is influential as much for what it says as for who said it. It was Richard Doll (along with Bradford Hill of the famous canons) who back in 1952 demonstrated the causal link between smoking and lung cancer, and the authority with which he has subsequently espoused the diet-disease thesis in relation to cancer has contributed enormously to its widespread acceptance.

The review 'estimates' that 30 per cent of cancers in the Western world are related to diet. The evidence is threefold, and comes from studies of precisely the kind cited in support of the diet-heart thesis. First are the 'cross-cultural studies', similar in method to Ancel Keys's Seven Country study. The report notes that 'the incidence of some cancers among people of a given age in different parts of the world varies by at least tenfold and sometimes a hundredfold'. Cancer of the oesophagus is 300 times more common in Iran than Nigeria; cancer of the lung is 35 times more common in Britain than Nigeria; cancer of the stomach is 25 times more common in Japan than Uganda, and cancer of the penis 300 times more common in Uganda than Israel. This wide variation in incidence suggests that there is something unique in the environment of one country compared with that of another which is responsible for the difference – the supposition being that in many instances 'something' is the type of food consumed.

Secondly, there are the migrant studies; the review observes: 'Evidence of a change in the incidence of cancer in a migrant group provides good evidence of the importance of lifestyle as one environmental factor in the production of disease.' The classic example (as with heart disease) is the change in rates of cancer in specific sites as Japanese migrants move from Japan to Hawaii to San Francisco. Here, however, the process goes both ways. In Japanese migrants to the US, the incidence of 'high-rate' Japanese cancers (of the oesophagus and stomach) falls towards the levels found in the US, while the incidence of 'low-rate' Japanese cancers (of the breast and colon) rises towards that found in the US. Once more, the inference is that Japanese patterns of disease change with a changing pattern of diet. And thirdly, there are studies which show that rates of specific cancers within one country rise and fall with time, strongly suggesting again that some external factor – such as food – induces the disease.

Doll and Peto go on to review the many possible mechanisms by which food might cause cancer. Cancer-inducing agents can indeed be found in food such as cycasin in the cycad nut and safrole in sassafras. Equally, however, there are elements in food which might protect against cancer – vitamin A is a strong candidate. However, none of these items of food have been shown to explain specific cancers. More interestingly, obese women have an increased risk of cancer of the womb, probably because the fat cells produce female hormones that can induce cancer – no 'overnutrition' can lead to cancer.

The classic example of the relationship between cancer and food remains that between fat consumption and breast cancer, already considered in Chapter 3. However, as will be recalled, it was not that fat in the diet directly causes the cancer, rather that in societies with a high fat intake, children grow rapidly, have an early puberty and a prolonged reproductive life during which the female hormones acting on the breast tissue can facilitate the development of cancer.

Doll and Peto's review appears as an intellectual *tour de force*, bringing together observations made over many years. But although the different rates of cancer between countries with different diets might be interpreted to mean that many cancers are diet-related, the actual number in which there are any demonstrable links is limited, and the links in any case appear to be indirect. Thus obesity may be related to cancer of the womb but obesity is not confined to those who eat a Western diet. Fat consumption can be linked with breast cancer, but this works indirectly through the prolongation of reproductive life. There is speculation that 'fibre deficiency' causes cancer of the colon. The statement that 30 per cent of cancers in the Western world are due to diet (with the implication that they could be prevented by a change of diet) was no more than a 'guesstimate' on the high side. Nonetheless it rapidly became an accepted part of the diet-disease orthodoxy that Doll and Peto had proved that at least 30 per cent (the more enthusiastic have suggested 70 per cent) of cancers are caused by the Western diet and can be prevented by appropriate dietary changes.

Lastly, it is worth noting that the emphasis on food minimises the most important determinant of cancer, which is age. About this Doll and Peto make an interesting comment:

> It is sometimes suggested that because cancer is a hundred times more likely to occur in any year in old people compared to the young, ageing *per se* should be thought of as an important determinant of cancer. We rather doubt whether this viewpoint is a scientifically fruitful one.

Not scientifically fruitful perhaps, but when considering the actual scope for the prevention of cancer, scientifically very important.

Dietary Fibre and Western Diseases

There is a reverse side to the argument that the Western diet causes Western diseases: namely, that the constituents of a Third World diet protect against those diseases. This is most dramatically seen by comparing the disease patterns of the peasant societies of sub-Saharan Africa with those of the Western world. In terms of health, these societies strongly resemble those of the West before the turn of the century, with high death rates among children and from infectious disease. But they are remarkably free from many contemporary Western ailments, including heart disease, strokes, cancers of the colon and breast, and inflammatory conditions of the gut such as appendicitis.

Being peasant societies, their major source of food is carbohydrate in the form of plants, roots and cereals. All of these are rich in 'dietary fibre', defined as 'any substance of plant origin which is not digested by the enzymes of the gut'. The suggestion therefore is that the relative paucity of these foods in the Western diet, and the consequent low-fibre intake of those living in the West, is an important cause of disease.[9]

The main evidence in favour of this thesis is again cross-cultural – that is, it is obtained by comparing the rates of different diseases in Africa and the West.

In the 1960s this observation was taken up and popularised by two British doctors, Denis Burkitt and Hugh Trowell, both of whom had worked for long periods in Africa. Burkitt, with the co-operation of a group of English schoolboys, started by examining how fibre in the diet influenced the quantity of the stool and the time it took to pass through the gut:

> After a lecture on health and food, I managed to enlist the help of thirty volunteers, who promised to swallow the pellets (to measure the time the stool took to pass through the bowel) and pass their stools into a plastic bag. They were to write their names and the time passed on labels and then deposit the bags in the school laboratory. I personally weighed the bags each morning for the next few days and carried them with me by train to London to be X-rayed in a hospital adjacent to my office.[10]

The results of the studies were published in 1972–3. The adult black population in rural Africa had stools weighing 300 to 500 grams which took 36 hours to pass. The comparable weight for the English schoolboys was 100 to 150 grams with transit times more than twice as long.

Such a significant difference in such an important area of human activity would be presumed to have some apparent effect. And certainly it is possible to hypothesise that not only might the bulky high-fibre stools cure constipation (certainly true), but also prevent bowel diseases such as appendicitis, diseases that might arise from straining when opening the bowels, varicose veins and piles. A more elaborate thesis is that they also prevent cancer of the colon, as heavy, rapid-transit stools minimise contact between potential cancer-inducing agents in the gut and the gut wall.

But whatever the hypotheses, it has never actually been possible to show that those people in the West who do get these diseases eat more or less fibre than anyone else in the West. Nor has it been possible to demonstrate that adopting a high-fibre diet will prevent them.

Salt and Hypertension

The evidence for a link between salt consumption and raised blood pressure (hypertension) leading to strokes derives from a similar pattern of cross-cultural studies already considered, although here the comparison is between 'primitive' societies (like Eskimos and

Aborigines) and the West rather than between specific countries.

The control of blood pressure is one of the most complex of all physiological mechanisms. It is influenced by an enormous number of stabilising systems, including nerves which monitor the pressure in the arteries, central mechanisms in the brain, the flux of calcium in and out of the walls of the arteries, a hormone secreted by the kidneys and others not yet discovered. It is possible to strip away one after another of these stabilising mechanisms and the control of the blood pressure remains steady.

The underlying cause of hypertension in which the blood pressure is continuously elevated remains unknown, but in view of the many complex physiological mechanisms involved it would seem unlikely that it should be anything as simple as an excess consumption of salt (not least because the body accurately regulates the amount of salt it needs, conserving it in the kidneys if the amount falls in the diet, excreting it in the urine if it is in abundance). Nonetheless the powerful imagery of excess salt consumption leading to raised blood pressure and hence to the subsequent risk of a stroke is, along with the diet-heart thesis, one of the most widely accepted nostrums of the diet-disease thesis.[11]

There certainly are 'primitive' populations in many parts of the world with low salt intakes and little or no hypertension, ranging from the Eskimos in the Arctic, through the Aborigines, to Pygmies and the inhabitants of the jungles of Papua New Guinea. And it is also certainly true that when they become Westernised their blood pressures tend to rise.

Within one country, however, the situation is predictably different: individuals with hypertension do not eat more salt than those without it. Furthermore, directly testing whether manipulation of the salt intake influences the blood pressure produces conflicting results. In people who already have hypertension, reducing salt consumption will reduce the blood pressure in some, but produces a paradoxical rise in others. In individuals with normal blood pressures only extreme manipulation of the salt intake seems to have any effect: massively reduce its quantity in the diet and the pressure might fall, massively overconsume and it might rise. So again, as with the other aspects of the diet-disease thesis, there is in fact no conclusive evidence or experimental proof to confirm the observations of the cross-cultural studies; and certainly none to incriminate salt consumption as a specific and preventable cause of high blood pressure and strokes.

*

The collective experience of the diet-heart thesis – the 30 per cent-of-cancers-attributable-to-diet thesis, the salt-hypertension thesis and the dietary fibre-diseases of the gut thesis – adds up to considerably more than its parts. It represents a package of ideas which are underlined by the notion that the 'affluent' West overconsumes, and that this overindulgence has lethal consequences. And with this comes the reverse side of the argument – that if Western man could get back to a 'less developed' pattern of food consumption (as found for example in Africa), he would be protected against disease. The antithesis is a powerful one.

But it does seem dependent on a deceptively powerful imagery of fat furring the arteries, salt overloading the circulation, fibre cleansing the bowel; images as powerful as those that once emphasised the virtue of dairy foods because they were 'high in bone- and flesh-forming material'. It raises the suspicion that the powerful incrimination of these foods is based on the simplicity of their message.

Furthermore, the logic of the thesis is dangerously near to being tautological: that is, some diseases occur in some countries because of the diet, and others in other countries because they have a different diet. It certainly seems naive simply to take the diseases common in the West, look around the world to find countries (or societies) where they are rare, and infer that the difference is due to patterns of food consumption. After all, the game can be played both ways. Forget about the 'diseases of civilisation' for a moment and concentrate on the Japanese. They have a high incidence of strokes and stomach cancer which declines when they move to the West – so by looking only at these diseases it is possible to demonstrate that Japanese migrants benefit from becoming Westernized. Equally, Africans are very vulnerable to infections, particularly tuberculosis and, more recently, AIDS, and have a high infant mortality rate: they might view with envy the position in the West where these problems are rare, and infer that a diet high in meat and dairy products protects against these diseases.

But even if the diet-disease thesis is correct, there remains the problem of the practical application of its insight. Should citizens of the West take a leaf out of the Japanese book and drastically reduce their dairy food consumption; or should they copy the New Guineans and abjure salt; or switch to cassava like the citizens of central Africa? What types of dietary changes are needed and how radical should they be? Radical changes are required to influence the biological functions of the body: is it realistic to suggest that people should make such changes? And if it is not realistic, why suggest them?

Despite these reservations and difficulties, many expert committees have been sufficiently impressed by the evidence cited above to recommend major changes in the Western diet. The most important question remains: are they right? After all, the evidence is essentially circumstantial – that is, if there were other explanations than patterns of food consumption for the different types of disease experienced by different countries or for the health experience of migrants, they would fit the data just as well. Certainly, compared to the quality of evidence that would confirm a causal relationship between food and disease, it is weak. It is one thing to point to the massive discrepancy, almost five hundredfold, in rates of beriberi between Javanese prisoners who eat polished and unpolished rice, and infer that beriberi might have something to do with removing the husk. It is quite another to point out that within the US, as the Framingham study showed, there is no difference in the fat consumption of those who do and do not get heart disease, and still to argue that fat consumption is an important cause of the disease.

In short, what is needed is more specific evidence of causality. And that means asking, like the engineer with his new model engine, does the thesis work? In scientific terms, it means submitting the theses to experiment and looking at the results. If *a* really does cause *b*, then changing *a* should change *b*. If fat really does cause heart disease, then changing the amount of fat in the diet should influence the subsequent risk of heart disease.

The diet-heart thesis has indeed been tested experimentally in the two ways it can be. The first is by taking a group of healthy men, encouraging them to reduce drastically the consumption of dairy foods and meat, and seeing if this reduces their subsequent incidence of heart disease. The second – and more interesting – is by looking at the changing pattern of heart disease over the last thirty years and seeing if it is paralleled by changing patterns of food consumption.

If the thesis is confirmed by these experiments, then there is no problem. Like curing beriberi with unpolished rice, or preventing lung cancer by not smoking, the knowledge that disease can be influenced by dietary changes could and should become part of common knowledge, and the guardians of the public health would be negligent if they were not to inform us accordingly (though what they might wish us to do with the knowledge is a different matter).

But if the thesis does not pass the test of experiment, that is important. It could mean that there is something deficient in the experiments themselves or it could mean that the circumstantial evidence is faulty and needs to be re-examined. We shall see.

8
The Evidence Tested

All the evidence presented in Chapter 7 for the diet-heart thesis – the comparison between countries of heart disease rates and severity of atherosclerosis, and the migrant studies – implicates the amount of fat in the diet as a cause of heart disease. It does not, however, provide positive proof that it *is* the cause, nor does it show that acting on this inference, by reducing the amount of fat in the diet, will reduce the rate of the disease. Aware of this defect in their case, the protagonists of the thesis set out in the early 1970s to remedy it in the only way possible: by mounting large experiments in which the efficacy of dietary changes could be tested by encouraging one group of people to change their diet, observing another group who did not and then comparing the eventual rates of heart disease in the two groups.

These experiments turned out to be the largest and most expensive ever conducted in the history of medicine. They took ten years to complete, involved over 60,000 men and cost in excess of £200 million. Their results are very important, because although the purpose was to provide proof of the thesis, they were in fact critically testing it. That is, failure to show that heart disease could be influenced by changes in diet would be an effective refutation of the thesis.

In all, five separate tests of the thesis were launched at this time. They can be divided conveniently into three groups.

1. Two trials involved middle-aged men with normal or near-normal levels of cholesterol in the blood: MRFIT (The Multiple Risk Factor Intervention Trial) in the US[1] and the WHO (World Health Organization) trial in five European countries.[2]

2. Two other trials also used healthy middle-aged men, but they had markedly elevated levels of cholesterol in the blood and so were

at increased risk of heart disease. These were the Oslo trial, in which attempts were made to lower the cholesterol by massive reductions in animal fat and meat in the diet, together with encouragement to give up smoking;[3] and the LRCCPPT (Lipid Research Clinics, Coronary Primary Prevention Trial) in which the intervention group were given a drug, cholestyramine, that lowers the level of cholesterol in the blood.[4]

3. The last test was not a trial in the accepted sense of the term, but a 'community-based heart disease prevention programme' in which the citizens of North Karelia, a province of Finland with a high rate of heart disease, were encouraged through the media and in a multiplicity of other ways to change their diet. The control group came from the neighbouring province of Kuopio.[5]

It is not necessary to describe the trials in detail other than to present the results, but the methods employed in the MRFIT and Oslo trials are of interest.

The MRFIT trial involved 12,000 men. Firstly, they were recruited into the project and all the risk factors considered important were identified. Next they were divided into two groups, balanced as far as possible in terms of age, smoking habits, raised blood pressure and level of cholesterol. Then one group was established as the intervention group, in which attempts were made to change the risk factors, whereas in the case of the other group – the control group – no attempts were made to change their lives. Close tabs were kept on all participants, their episodes of illness monitored and causes of death established.

The intervention itself took the following forms. Those in the intervention group were started with an intensive integrated effort to stop smoking and change their diet. After this, individual counselling to back up the message was provided every four months by an intervention team headed by a behavioural scientist and including nutritionists, nurses, physicians and health educators. The intervention focused on modifying the three risk factors for heart disease. Those with hypertension were treated with drugs, and smokers were exposed to 'conventional behaviour modification techniques', supported by aversion therapy and hypnosis. Finally, in an attempt to influence the level of blood cholesterol, the intervention teams sought 'to encourage the development of life-long shopping, cooking and eating patterns' designed to reduce the amount of fat in the diet. This meant drinking skimmed milk, abjuring cream, using margarine as a spread, eating only low-fat cheeses, restricting eggs to one or two per week, avoiding all rich cakes, puddings and pastries, and considerably reducing the amount of meat consumed. If food was an important cause of heart disease, then by the end of the experiment the incidence of the disease in the intervention group would be lower than in the control group.

For the intervention group in the Oslo trial the dietary changes were spelt out more specifically: no milk, butter, cream or high-fat cheeses; eggs restricted to one per week, no sausage, salami or other high-fat meats; fish and vegetable fillings for sandwiches, and reduction of sweet drinks and alcohol.

All the trials ran for the best part of a decade and the results were reported in succession from 1981 to 1984. They were remarkably consistent in their verdict on the diet-heart thesis (Table 8.1). At the end of the MRFIT and WHO trials there was *no difference* in the rates of heart disease between the intervention and control groups. By contrast, intervention in the Oslo and LRCCPPT trials, where the men had very high cholesterol levels, did reduce the rate of heart disease back to that of the rest of the population, although there was *no difference* in overall mortality rates between the two groups. In the North Karelia project there was *no difference* in the rates of heart disease between North Karelia and the control province of Kuopio, although each province had less heart disease than had been predicted.

The results are very instructive. The changes in diet recommended for the intervention groups were radical, as they had to be to hope to influence the level of cholesterol in the blood. They can be used to illustrate the scale of changes in diet that would have had to have occurred in the West over the last thirty years if the epidemic of heart disease were to be attributable to increasing fat consumption.

They confirm that a high cholesterol level in the blood is a causative risk factor for heart disease by demonstrating that lowering it (whether by drugs or by diet) reduces the incidence of heart disease.

However, and most importantly, they show that encouraging those with normal cholesterol levels to reduce the amount of fat in their diets does not influence the subsequent risk of the disease. That is, fat consumption in itself is not a determinant cause of heart disease.

There is another way of critically testing the thesis, and that is to examine whether changing patterns of heart disease in different

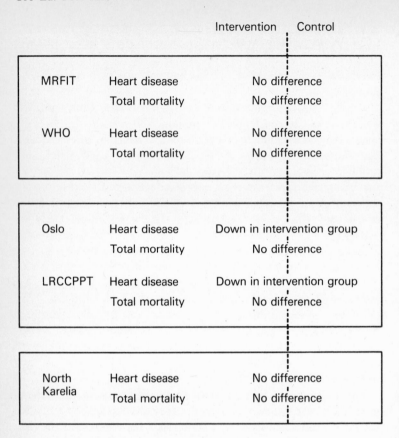

Table 8.1 *Results of the major trials*

countries over the last thirty years have been reflected in changing patterns of food consumption.

This is possible because in 1968, just as all the scientific evidence was being accumulated to indict the Western diet in heart disease, a very unexpected thing happened. After a relentless rise over forty years, mortality rates started to fall in the US in all classes, all ethnic and all age groups, and continued to fall year by year in an almost exact reversal of the pattern of its previous ascendancy. Even more remarkably, at exactly the same time and at the same rate, heart disease started to decline simultaneously in several other countries. Now, if fat consumption is a cause of heart disease, this change in the pattern should be reflected in changes in patterns of food consumption. That this is a legitimate test of the thesis is proved by the historical analogy of alcohol consumption and deaths from liver cirrhosis.

Although alcohol is not the only cause of liver cirrhosis, it is far and away the most important, so one would expect during periods when its consumption is restricted that there should be a marked reduction in deaths from the disease, and this is indeed the case. There have been several periods when the consumption of alcohol has markedly declined, in the US during Prohibition, and in France and Britain during the Second World War.[6] The example from Paris is the most dramatic. Here alcohol was restricted to half a litre per week not only for the war years, but right up to 1948. The fall in mortality from liver cirrhosis exactly coincides with this period of rationing. A similar picture is seen in the US during Prohibition, although the persistence of deaths from the disease during this period is a testament to the degree of evasion. Finally in England and Wales, there is a remarkable parallelism over the last fifty years (see Fig. 8.1), between alcohol consumption and liver cirrhosis which as in France falls most precipitately during the war years.

With this analogy fresh in the mind, it is appropriate to look again at the changing pattern of premature heart disease in the US and neighbouring countries, Australia, Canada and New Zealand over the last thirty years (shown at the top of the graph in Fig. 8.2). The contrast could not be more striking.[7] Whereas the liver cirrhosis graph fluctuates in a way that would be consistent with a disease caused by a social phenomenon such as the consumption of alcohol, that of heart disease is virtually straight up and down, with its peak in 1968. So in order to explain the changing pattern of the disease in terms of changes in diet, it is necessary to presuppose that in not one, but several countries, the citizens simultaneously, consistently and steadily made major changes in diet, first by markedly increasing their consumption of animal fats and then by decreasing it. This would seem unlikely. So what have been the changes in food consumption patterns?

This is not as straightforward as observing the changes in heart disease rates because the reliability of the available data on food consumption is uncertain. Furthermore, it is expressed in terms of 'total' fat, and so does not distinguish between 'saturated' and 'polyunsaturated' fats; and finally, it involves comparing food consumption figures for a whole country with the pattern of disease in one group of the population, middle-aged males. These are inescapable weaknesses, but it is permissible to use the data for

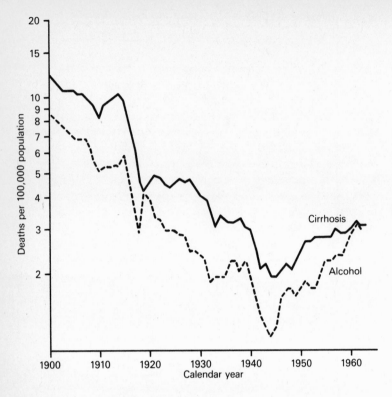

Fig.8.1 *Death rate from cirrhosis of the liver in the U.K. closely parallels the national consumption of alcohol*

two reasons. Because such major dietary changes are needed to influence the level of blood cholesterol, the exact figures are less important than seeing whether there are major trends in one direction or another. Secondly, there is no reason to suppose that the pattern of food consumption in middle-aged males should be any different from that of the rest of the population.

According to the data, then, fat consumption (shown at the bottom of Fig. 8.2) appears to have remained relatively stable over the last thirty years. It certainly does not parallel the changing pattern of heart disease.[8] Unlike the liver cirrhosis analogy, the pattern of heart disease does not resemble a disease that could be caused by a social factor, and the consumption of the presumed cause of the disease bears no relation to the disease itself. Of special interest is the experience of Japan in the left-hand corner of the

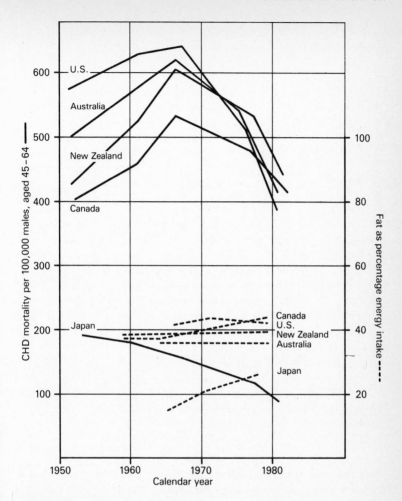

Fig.8.2 *Heart disease (CHD) mortality rate per 100,000 males aged 45–64 compared with trends in fat consumption for the U.S., Australia, New Zealand, Canada and Japan*

graph. It has always had a low rate of heart disease, yet despite increasing Westernisation of the diet over the last thirty years, with a rise in fat consumption of over 50 per cent, the rates of the disease have not risen.

It is perhaps surprising to observe that the total amount of fat in the diet of the average US citizen has not changed much over the last three decades. Exposed to the full blast of the diet-heart thesis they might have been expected to reduce their consumption of dairy foods particularly over the last decade. And in fact they have. The consumption of milk, eggs and butter have all fallen, but this has been compensated by a marked increase in meat consumption during the same period, so the amount of fat in the diet has changed little.[9]

The failure to demonstrate parallelism in the US and neighbouring countries is damning in itself, and is further reinforced by considering heart disease in other countries. Even more interesting things begin to happen when the global pattern of heart disease is examined.

Looking first at the countries of Eastern Europe, it appears that heart disease has been rising exponentially over the last fifteen years in a similar way to that experienced by the US and neighbouring countries in the 1950s and early 1960s (Fig. 8.3).

In the countries of Western Europe, on the other hand, there appears to be a pattern of heart disease intermediate between that of the US and the countries of the Soviet bloc. The rise in heart disease in the 1960s, continues in Sweden, has been followed by a fall in Finland, by the beginnings of a decline in England and Wales, and by little change in Italy (Fig. 8.4).

Again there appears to be no parallel between heart disease and food consumption patterns, at least in Western Europe. The figures for Eastern Europe are unavailable except for Yugoslavia, which of all the examples cited is the only one where there is a possible parallel between fat consumption and heart disease.

The experience of some of the countries deserves a little further elaboration. Japan and Italy featured in Ancel Keys's Seven Country study and were particularly important in showing that low intakes of saturated fat were associated with low rates of heart disease. Both countries have subsequently experienced increasing Westernization of their diets with rising fat consumption, but there has not been the predicted rise in incidence of the disease. Then there is the contrasting experience of the US and Sweden. Both are considered 'health-conscious countries' and might be expected to have reduced their consumption of fat. Not only is this not apparent, but they have had exactly contrary experiences of heart disease – in the US falling dramatically, in Sweden continuing to rise. Finally Finland, which at one time had the highest rate of heart disease in the world, has had its fall, accompanied, if this data is reliable, by a paradoxical small rise in fat consumption.

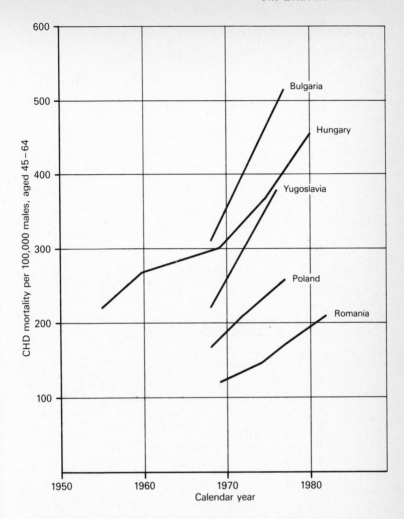

Fig.8.3 *Heart disease (CHD) mortality rate per 100,000 males aged 45 – 64 in Hungary, Bulgaria, Yugoslavia, Poland and Romania*

Might there be other explanations? After all, heart disease is 'multifactorial'; that is, many risk factors have been associated with it. But this only makes the pattern of the disease even more difficult to explain, because it would presuppose that the populations of different countries simultaneously not only altered their diets (which ostensibly they have not), but also in concert changed such

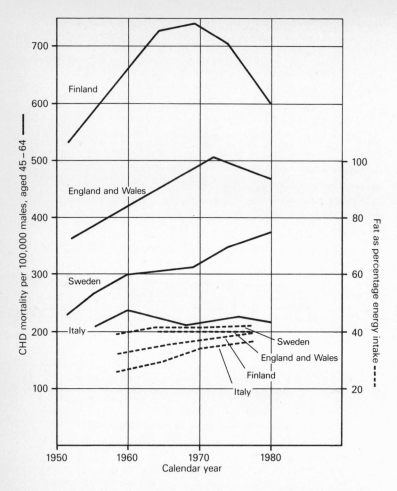

Fig.8.4 *Heart disease (CHD) mortality rate per 100,000 males aged 45–64 compared with trends in fat consumption for selected countries in Western Europe*

other lifestyle factors as smoking, exercise, stress and blood pressure.

The lack of parallelism between heart disease and food consumption is immensely important, and taken with the results of the trials would appear completely to refute the diet-heart thesis. But we can go further than this negative conclusion, because a look at the global pattern of heart disease also points to a possible alternative explanation.

It appears from the data that heart disease is slowly moving from West to East across the developed world, although affecting some countries more seriously than others. In addition to the geographical pattern, there is a temporal one. The rise in heart disease in Western Europe followed that in the US by ten years. Now heart disease is rising in Eastern Europe, lagging behind that of Western Europe. If this geographical and temporal pattern reflected a deeper underlying pattern of the disease, one would expect to see the same phenomenon across a large country like the US – i.e., the pattern of the disease moving from West to East. And such a pattern does indeed exist. The decline in heart disease in the US first started on the Western seaboard in 1955, and then over the next ten years slowly moved across the country. The beginning of the decline on the West coast preceded by a decade the overall decline in the US.[10]

What to make of this? We have been so conditioned to believing that heart disease is caused by 'unhealthy lifestyles', and yet it is inconceivable to suggest that a disease exhibiting such a marked rise and fall within one country, and with such a definite geographical shift, is compatible with this explanation. Rather it suggests the underlying cause of heart disease is an unknown biological factor – a factor X – that originated in the 1920s, wreaked its havoc for three decades, and then exhausted itself.

So how, then, to explain the fact that there are obvious risk factors for the disease such as smoking, raised blood pressure and high cholesterol levels in the blood? How to explain the different incidence of the disease between countries? It is possible that the identified risk factors are additional but not determinant factors in the disease. When factor X is in the ascendant, it falls most heavily on those who smoke a lot, or who have very high levels of cholesterol in the blood. Equally it is possible that factor X falls most heavily on countries with a lot of meat and dairy fat in the diet – countries with higher levels of cholesterol than those with less fat, and so suffering more severe atherosclerosis (as the international comparison of atherosclerosis showed). But here again diet is additional rather than determinant, just as smoking is an additional but not determinant cause of death from Legionnaire's disease.

If the amount of fat in the diet is not a direct cause of heart disease rather than a direct cause, it should be that within one country (rather than comparing different countries) the evidence linking fat intake to the disease will fail to fulfil Bradford Hill's crucial canons of proof. Let us make the test.

Is the thesis biologically plausible? No. It is superficially an attractive notion that fat in the diet affects the severity of athero-sclerosis by influencing the level of cholesterol in the blood and thus leads to heart disease. This, after all, is the basis of the common belief that fat in the diet furs up the arteries. But we have seen it requires major alterations in the amount of meat and dairy foods in the diet to change the level of cholesterol in the blood. The changing pattern of the disease would therefore have required major changes in the consumption of these foods, and these changes have not occurred.

Does the amount of fat in the diet predict the subsequent risk of heart disease? No. As the Framingham study showed, those with heart disease do not consume more fat than those without the disease.

Does a high intake of fat lead to the high cholesterol level found in those at high risk for heart disease? No. The high cholesterol levels in these individuals is related to an abnormality of the protein that transports cholesterol in the blood, and not to the amount of fat in the diet.

Is there a dose-response relationship as with smoking and lung cancer; that is, do increasing amounts of fat in the diet predictably increase the risk of the disease? No. The Framingham study fails to show that the more fat in the diet, the higher the risk of the disease.

Does the supposed relationship hold over time – is the incidence of the disease paralleled by changing patterns of fat consumption? Again the answer is no.

Finally, there is the definitive experiment: does reducing the amount of fat in the diet reduce the incidence of the disease? No. The trials show this is not the case, with the exception of those with very high levels of cholesterol in the blood.

The diet-heart thesis fulfils none of Bradford Hill's canons of proof. It stands refuted, and the link, if there is one, must be indirect.

But it has also been possible to identify a unifying biological cause for the disease which explains all aspects of the evidence that the diet-heart thesis cannot accommodate. It explains why there is no relationship between fat intake and the subsequent risk of heart disease within one country. It explains why it is possible to die from heart disease with little or no atherosclerosis in the arteries. It explains why it is not possible to demonstrate parallelism between heart disease rates and changing patterns of fat consumption; why the rate of heart disease in Japan has remained constant despite increasing Westernisation of the diet; why the rate of the disease continues to rise in very health-conscious countries such as Sweden. And, finally, it explains why the trials failed.

If fat consumption is only indirectly involved in heart disease as an associative or additional factor, that means there must be something wrong with the circumstantial evidence in favour of the diet-heart hypothesis, something wrong with the cross-cultural comparisons, the migrant studies and so on, all of which inferred a direct causal link. So it is time now to re-examine that evidence. It will not turn out to be false in itself; but a look at it from a different perspective, with the addition of further 'omitted' data, shows that it does not demonstrate what is claimed for it.

9
Flaws in the Argument

The diet-heart thesis employs five different sources of evidence to suggest that there is a direct causal link between diet and heart disease: the comparison between countries (the cross-cultural studies); the experience of migrants; the international comparison of the severity of atherosclerosis in the coronary arteries; the low levels of heart disease among vegetarian Seventh Day Adventists; and the decline of heart disease in certain countries during the Second World War. However, as we have seen, the inference of a causal relationship is false because the thesis fails to fulfil Bradford Hill's canons and has been refuted by experiment. Re-examination of those sources of evidence will therefore demonstrate that they are flawed.

The Cross-cultural Studies

Ancel Keys's Seven Country study showed that between countries there was an apparent step-like progression in the amount of saturated fat in the diet and the incidence of heart disease from Japan at one extreme to Finland at the other.[1] It is perhaps doubtful whether the experience of Japanese fishermen is really comparable to that of US railroaders and Finnish lumberjacks, but this is not a very useful line of enquiry.

Start with adding more countries to the seven in Keys's study and what happens (Fig. 9.1)?[2] This still leaves Japan with the lowest rates at one end and the Finnish with the highest at the other; but what is more striking is that for a given amount of fat in the diet – between 35 and 40 per cent of total energy intake – the heart disease rates varies fivefold, from 200 per 100,000 in France to 1,000 per

100,000 in Finland. Here the comparison between countries fails to demonstrate a causal relationship between fat and the disease, because it fails to explain the France–Finland difference. Keys's study is therefore suspect firstly because it relies on a very selective group of countries.

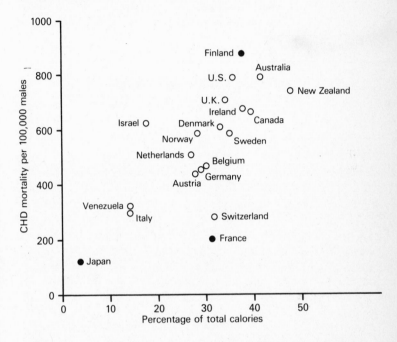

Fig.9.1 *When similar countries are compared (France and Finland) there is no relationship between the amount of meat and dairy products (as a percentage of total calories in the diet and the rate of heart disease)*

But even if Keys had not been so selective, it would still be inadmissible to use comparisons between countries in support of the thesis, for the following reason. There are two aspects to be taken into consideration when thinking about why an individual succumbs to a disease. The first is exposure to the cause (if it is known), and the second is the individual's susceptibility to that cause. Not everyone who is exposed to the tuberculosis bacillus gets tuberculosis, not everyone who smokes gets lung cancer. It is a primary assumption of the cross-cultural studies, however, that any cause, in this case food, has the same effect on inducing a disease, irrespective of the cultural and ethnic composition of those who are exposed to it. Only on this condition can a comparison between countries demonstrate that increasing consumption of fat is causally related to increasing rates of heart disease. But is this assumption correct? Do different populations have the same susceptibility to a given cause of a disease?

Consider a disease in which the cause is known: smoking and lung cancer. If the only consideration in the incidence of a disease were its cause and the susceptibility of a population was unimportant, it should be possible to demonstrate the type of cross-cultural correlation between smoking and lung cancer as Keys showed for fat and heart disease. But it is not. Cross-cultural studies do not indicate a relation between countries of the amount smoked and the incidence of lung cancer. For a given national consumption of cigarettes per head of population, the rates of lung cancer vary fivefold between Mexico and Belgium (Fig. 9.2).[3,4]

Keys's Seven Country study shows why. If the US and Northern European countries are together compared with the countries around the Mediterranean – Greece, Yugoslavia and Italy – it is possible to show that within these groups smoking causes lung cancer; that is, with increasing consumption of cigarettes there is an increasing risk of the disease. However, there is a marked difference in the amount of lung cancer found for the same amount of cigarettes smoked (Fig. 9.3). Keys does not give the data for the Japanese, but their incidence of lung cancer is still lower than that of the Greeks and Italians even though they too are heavy smokers. One might think of explanations for this difference in experience of the disease – perhaps they smoke different types of cigarettes in Japan and around the Mediterranean, or perhaps there is less pollution. But the realistic explanation must be that a collection of various factors, genetic, cultural and environmental, means that the Japanese and Mediterranean peoples are less susceptible to the disease than Americans and North Europeans, even though smoking remains the determinant cause. And as the populations of these different countries have different susceptibilities to the given cause of lung cancer, simply comparing them cannot in itself show that the more cigarettes smoked, the higher the rate of lung cancer.

On the other hand, comparing countries of roughly similar cultural and ethnic constitution and so presumably similar susceptibilities, like the countries of the Western world, demonstrates that a cross-cultural correlation between smoking and lung cancer does hold (Fig. 9.4).[5]

So if cross-cultural comparisons are to be used, it is only legiti-

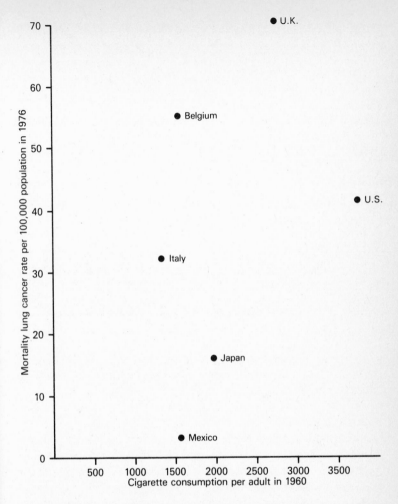

Fig.9.2 *There is no relationship between cigarette smoking and death rate from lung cancer between countries*

mate to employ comparisons between roughly similar societies. In the case of the diet-heart thesis, the comparison between roughly similar societies such as France and Finland, which does not show a correlation, is therefore admissible. By contrast, Keys's study, even if he had not chosen such a highly selected group of countries to prove his point, would still be inadmissible because it relies on a comparison between such diverse societies.

The exception that proves this rule is the correlation between

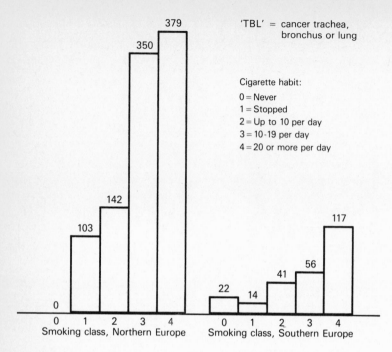

Fig.9.3 *Within both Northern and Southern Europe the risk of lung cancer rises with increased cigarette smoking, but the risk is much greater in Northern Europe*

breast cancer and fat intake which holds both between roughly similar countries and very diverse ones, because here fat intake first has to lengthen the duration of reproductive life before it can influence the risk of the disease.

Keys's cross-cultural study cannot therefore be adduced as evidence in favour of the thesis, because it relies on an overwhelmingly partial selection of countries to fit the hypothesised relationship between fat and heart disease (if he had looked at other countries he would not have been able to demonstrate it), and on a false assumption that people from very different ethnic and cultural backgrounds have the same susceptibility to a given cause of disease.

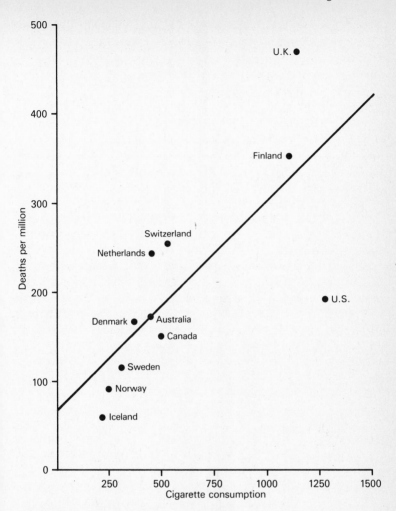

Fig.9.4 *When similar countries are compared there is a relationship between cigarette smoking and the death rate from lung cancer*

The Migrant Studies

The second source of evidence in favour of the diet-heart thesis is the migrant studies, in which the rate of heart disease increases in Japanese migrants as they move to the US.[6] The proposition is that this can be attributed to increasing amounts of fat in the diet.

The most interesting way of testing this suggestion is to look at the experience of another group of migrants from a country with the same type of diet as the US but a lower rate of heart disease. If the inference about fat is correct, then their rates of heart disease should remain low when they move to the US – but they do not. The migrants from Sweden with a lower rate of heart disease than the US increase their rates of heart disease on migration even though their dietary patterns change little.[7] So whatever does cause the rise in heart disease of Japanese migrants, it is not what they eat. One can see this better by looking again at the exception that proves the rule – breast cancer and fat intake. The incidence of breast cancer rises in the children of Japanese migrants to the US in line with increasing fat consumption, but stays the same in children of Swedish migrants for whom the amount of fat in the diet remains the same as in the country of origin.[8,9]

What other explanation can there be for the rising rate of heart disease among Japanese migrants to the US? The answer is to be found by looking at the totality of changes in the diseases from which they suffer. The Japanese have very high rates of death from stroke and of cancer of the stomach, and low rates for heart disease and cancers of the breast and colon. As they move to the US, this pattern of disease is totally reversed; that is, they lose Japanese-style diseases and acquire US-style diseases (Fig. 9.5). A similar effect can be shown for migrants to Britain from countries as diverse as Ireland, Poland, Italy and the Caribbean, over a whole range of diseases such as cancers of the lung and cervix, strokes and heart disease. In each case, whether the disease rate is initially lower or higher in the country of origin than in Britain, the rate of disease in migrants tends towards that found in Britain.[10]

So it is a generalised phenomenon that migrants lose the pattern of disease of their home country and acquire that of their adopted country. Even without the experience of the Swedes to show that the changing pattern of heart disease of the Japanese cannot be due to changing dietary patterns, it would still not be admissible to use the experience of the Japanese migrants as specific evidence in favour of the thesis. This is because it involves extrapolating from a generalised phenomenon (that migrants will suffer less from the diseases of their country of origin and more from those of the adopted country) to infer a specific causal relationship (that the rise in heart disease in Japanese migrants to the US is due to a change in diet).

The uselessness of the migrant studies to illustrate a causal

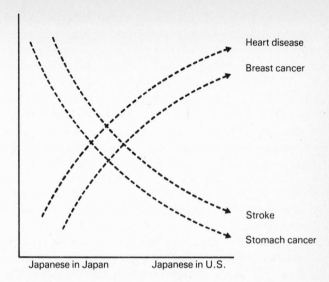

Fig.9.5 *Changing trends of diseases in Japanese migrants to the United States*

relationship between food and disease is obvious because they can be used to infer whatever thesis one wishes. By focusing on the falling rates of stroke and cancer of the stomach in Japanese migrants to the US, for example, it is equally possible to argue that increased fat intake is beneficial.

The changing pattern of disease among migrants is tantalising evidence that these diseases are environmentally determined, but that gets us no nearer defining *which* feature of the environment. We can however show that it is not food by comparing the pattern of the disease with patterns of food consumption within one country.

In Japan and the West there have been two broad dietary patterns over the last fifty years. In Western countries the diet has remained relatively stable with a constant amount of fat, whereas in Japan it has become increasingly Westernised with increasing amounts of fat. Therefore if the Western diet were an important cause of disease, they would have remained relatively stable in the West but have increased in Japan. If the Japanese diet were an important cause of diseases, they would have declined in Japan as its diet has become Westernised. Fig. 9.6 shows what in fact has happened.

Stroke is an example. It has been declining in Japan with increasing Westernisation,[11] and declines in Japanese migrants to the US; evidence that it is caused by the traditional Japanese diet and by the benefits of increasing fat consumption? No, because it has also been declining in the West where dietary patterns have remained stable.[12] The same arguments apply to stomach cancer, declining in Japan,[13] and in Japanese migrants to the US, but not due to the traditional Japanese diet because also declining in the West.[14] Then premature heart disease, stable in Japan despite Westernisation and declining in the West though dietary patterns are stable. It certainly is not due to fat consumption. And finally, the exception that proves the rule. Breast cancer, rising in Japan with increasing fat in the diet,[15] but stable in the West; rising in Japanese migrants to the US, but stable in migrants from countries with Western diets on moving to the US.

This gets us no further in explaining why diseases rise or fall in migrants or why they rise and fall within one country, but it does at least allow us to exonerate food as their cause (except indirectly for fats and breast cancer).

What can we conclude? That different countries have different types of age-related illness. That the causes of these diseases might be environmentally determined because their incidence changes on migration and fluctuates with time; but that it is not possible to implicate any specific aspect of the diet (except for fat consumption and breast cancer), firstly because the incidence of diseases in migrants moving between countries with similar diets changes as much as in those moving between countries of very different dietary patterns; and secondly because diseases rise and fall within one country with no relation to the dietary patterns of those countries. Even if we could show that food was an important cause of these illnesses and suggested that everyone changed their diet, the Japanese to a Western-style diet and vice versa, the overall result would only be an exchange of one pattern of disease for another.

The Seventh Day Adventists

The low rate of heart disease among the vegetarian Seventh Day Adventists is frequently cited as evidence in favour of the thesis – although they also tend to have lower rates of a wide variety of diseases not usually attributed to fat consumption, which suggests again that the statistics are only part of a generalised phenomenon.[16] The way to test this piece of evidence is to look at a similar

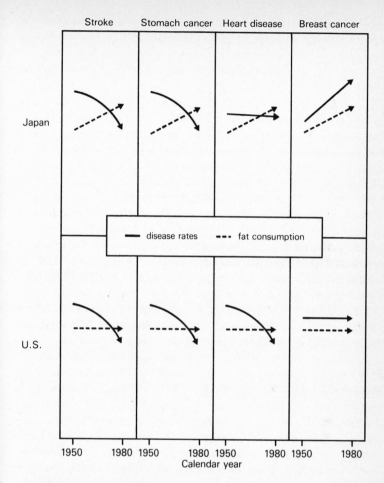

Fig.9.6 *Changing patterns of stroke, stomach cancer, heart disease and breast cancer contrasted with changing dietary patterns in Japan and the West, 1950 – 1980*

group of people, a highly religious, tightly knit community like the Mormons, who are meat and dairy food consumers. If the diet-heart thesis is correct, they should have a higher rate of heart disease than the Seventh Day Adventists, similar indeed to that of the rest of the US population. Interestingly, however, Mormons too have low rates of heart disease and cancer.[17] The evidence from the Adventists is testament to the power of prayer, not to the role of diet in heart disease.

The War Years

Even if the famine and deprivation of the war years were to have produced a decline in heart disease, it is questionable how useful this insight would be as the type of dietary restrictions experienced then are scarcely suitable to recommend to civilian populations during peacetime. The fall in mortality is nonetheless impressive, but it is above all the rise in heart disease amongst middle-aged men that requires an explanation, and it is the mortality rates of this group that needs to be focused upon. Here, needless to say, the picture is different. The numbers of deaths in all age groups attributed to atherosclerosis did indeed fall, as the diet-heart thesis protagonists emphasise; but heart disease in middle-aged men continued to rise in Britain during the war years despite a major reduction in fat consumption.[18] Examining in more detail the figures for Norway reveals that the mortality rates for premature heart disease altered little during the war years.[19]

Atherosclerosis

Finally, there is the evidence from the International Atherosclerosis Project, that atherosclerosis in coronary artery specimens from different countries appears to be most severe in those countries with the highest rates of heart disease. If the 'epidemic' of premature heart disease over the last fifty years is due to dietary-induced changes in cholesterol, leading to increasing severity of atherosclerosis, then over the period that heart disease has been increasing atherosclerosis will have become more severe in Western countries. But in fact the changing pattern of heart disease has not been paralleled by major changes in fat consumption sufficient to influence the level of cholesterol and through that the severity of atherosclerosis. And again, there is no relation between the rise in heart disease and increasing severity of atherosclerosis.

J. N. Morris of the Medical Research Council analysed the data on severity of atherosclerosis in autopsy specimens from the London Hospital over twenty-five years from 1915 to the outbreak of the Second World War, that is, over the period that heart disease was beginning to 'take off' in Britain. He found that the severity of atherosclerosis actually *decreased* during this period, but that there was an increase in the number of cases where the coronary arteries were occluded by thrombus and where there was evidence of having had a heart attack. He commented subsequently:

> Coronary occlusion (i.e. the blockage of the coronary arteries) occurs on the basis of coronary atherosclerosis, but over and above that other causes are importantly involved in producing the occlusion, causes unrelated to atherosclerosis. Atherosclerosis is only an element, it is a necessary but not sufficient cause.[20]

A similar study comparing the extent of atherosclerosis with rates of heart disease in similar countries led to the same conclusion. In this case the comparison was between Glasgow and Greater London. For middle-aged men, heart disease mortality is twice as high in Glasgow than London; but the amount of atherosclerosis and the severity of narrowing of the coronary arteries is the reverse – greater in London than Glasgow.[21]

The evidence from the studies of the severity of atherosclerosis in different countries would therefore point to the conclusion already arrived at, that atherosclerosis might contribute to the seriousness of heart disease but is not a determinant cause.

Examination of the circumstantial evidence for the diet-heart thesis leaves it rather forlorn. It has been possible to exclude the cross-cultural studies because they rely on a selective comparison of very diverse cultures; and the Japanese migrant studies because they are countered by the experience of the Swedish migrants, and because it is anyway a generalised phenomenon that migrants change their pattern of disease. The experience of the vegetarian Adventists has been countered by that of the Mormons, the evidence from the war years by closer examination of the statistics for middle-aged men, and the comparison of severity of atherosclerosis between countries by showing that over time the increasing rates of heart disease have not been paralleled by increasing severity of atherosclerosis. So the refutation of the thesis, its failure to fulfil Bradford Hill's canons and the negative results of the critical experiments, are entirely predictable because the evidence in favour of the thesis is found on close examination to be completely flawed.

Nonetheless, it remains true that the disease is commonest in those with high levels of cholesterol in the blood and is much commoner in Western countries than elsewhere. So even if fat consumption is not a primary cause of the disease, it might be a necessary or secondary cause in that it falls most heavily on countries with relatively high fat diets and so relatively more severe atherosclerosis. This leaves the question of whether the consumption of saturated fat should be drastically reduced, hoping thereby to reduce the severity of atherosclerosis and 'contain' the epidemic in this way.

We have already come across some of the answers to this question. Firstly, it is unlikely to be effective: it would be like trying to prevent death from Legionnaire's disease by discouraging smoking rather than identifying the bacterium that causes the disease and reducing people's exposure to it. Secondly, it is very difficult to influence the level of cholesterol in the blood by dietary changes; only major reductions in fat intake are effective and even then the result is uncertain with large variation of response between individuals. It would thus be very difficult to promote the necessary dietary changes in the general population. As the programme of trials demonstrates, enormous efforts have to be made to change long-held cultural habits of food consumption, and it would be wrong to promote such changes if they were unlikely to be successful. Thirdly, if the decline in heart disease in the US and other countries is anything to go by, the disease is already in decline and there is no reason to believe that Western Europe should not follow the pattern of the US. By the time enough young people have been encouraged radically to alter their diets sufficiently to influence the severity of atherosclerosis, the disease could well be a thing of the past. Finally, changes in dietary patterns could have unforeseen consequences. It has already been observed that major restrictions of fat consumption might restrict growth and curtail the length of women's reproductive life.

But actually the putative dangers of radically reducing fat consumption lie closer to home, and involve one final example of how a one-sided examination of evidence can distort reality.

The danger of having a very high level of cholesterol in the blood is that it increases the risk of heart disease. But are there any dangers from a low blood cholesterol? Looking at the total death rates at different levels of cholesterol, they appear to be lowest at the 'mean' or average cholesterol, the level of cholesterol most frequently found in the population. But the total death rate then slowly rises on either side of the mean, increasing in those with increasingly high levels of cholesterol because of its effect on heart disease, but also increasing in those with decreasingly low cholesterol levels. As those with high cholesterol are at high risk of heart disease, it appears that those with low cholesterols are at high risk of other diseases, particularly cancer.[22] So if the suggestion is (as it is) that everyone should reduce their level of fat in the diet in order to achieve lower cholesterol levels and therefore less severe atherosclerosis, the unhappy consequence might be to increase the risk of cancer in that large section of the population with normal cholesterol levels.

This uncomfortable observation has been a subject of some embarrassment to the diet-heart protagonists because it implies that radical changes in the nation's diet sufficient to lower everyone's cholesterol level would increase the likelihood of getting cancer, if the low cholesterol–high cancer risk relationship were causal. Their response is that it is not, but rather that the low cholesterol levels found in those who subsequently develop cancer are caused by the cancer somehow lowering the levels of cholesterol in the blood.[23] This is a consoling possibility, but one can't be sure; and if reducing high cholesterol levels reduces the risk of heart disease, it is at least a possibility that lowering normal cholesterol levels will increase the risk of cancer.

And so it has come to this, the simple message that 'cutting down on fat will reduce heart disease' would have an insignificant effect because fat consumption is only indirectly related to the disease, would require changes in diet that in practical terms could not possibly be implemented by the public, and if they were implemented would carry unknown dangers.

Turning to other components of the diet-disease thesis, it is not appropriate to attempt to refute them each in turn, as the same arguments apply as with the diet-heart thesis; namely, that the circumstantial evidence in favour of the separate theses from the cross-cultural and migrant studies is inadmissible, while the application of Bradford Hill's canons of epidemiological proof to the evidence for the relationship between these diseases and their supposed dietary cause produces only negative results.

Diet and Cancer

In their very influential review, Sir Richard Doll and Richard Peto argued that '30 per cent of cancers are diet-related', although the reasons for arriving at this exact figure are not given and it has all the appearance of having been plucked out of the air. The evidence they cite depends overwhelmingly on cross-cultural and migrant studies, but contains the seeds of refutation of its own inference, as by showing that there are high-incidence cancers in many different societies and that the changes on migration apply to all these cancers (rare cancers becoming commoner, common cancers becoming rarer), suggesting that cancer is an inescapable part of the human condition, and that the only effect of trying to prevent them by dietary means (if they were to be related to food) would be to exchange one lot of cancers for another. There are no societies in which cancer is not a common cause of death.

The exceptions to this observation have already been noted. Obesity may lead to cancer of the womb, because fat cells produce female hormones that can induce cancer, but this cannot be used to indict the Western diet in particular as one can find obesity in any society. As for breast cancer and fat consumption, we have confronted the practical problems of trying to apply this knowledge to prevent the disease.

Dietary Fibre and Western Diseases

The fibre thesis is relevant to the treatment of constipation but there seems to be no reason why those who do not suffer from this complaint should go on a high-fibre diet merely for the sake of having bulky, loose stools. Its links with other diseases remain speculative; varicose veins and piles are meant to be related to straining at stool, but is there any evidence that those suffering from these diseases suffer more from constipation than those who do not? No. One study in Scandinavia showed that the amount of one type of fibre in the diet, pentose, related to the incidence of colon cancer,[24] but elsewhere no one has been able to show that those who get the disease eat more or less fibre than anyone else. The dietary fibre thesis illustrates how a plausible idea can fade on closer examination.

Salt and Hypertension

The supposed link between salt and hypertension is heavily dependent on the comparison between 'underdeveloped' societies and the Western world, and the observation that 'acculturation' of these peoples is accompanied by a rise in blood pressure. Leaving aside the obvious point that salt is not the only distinguishing feature in this comparison, again there is nothing to suggest that those who get hypertension in the West eat more salt than those who do not. Finally, if salt were an important cause one would expect that manipulating the salt intake should influence the blood pressure. As seen, this will only happen at extremes of consumption and even then the result is unpredictable, widely variable and can, when severely restricted, lead to a paradoxical rise in blood pressure.

Now it is possible to see the fragility of the overall thesis: how heavily dependent it is on unwarranted inferences from a one-sided presentation of facts, and how much it relies both on the powerful imagery of imagined mechanisms of disease and on a politicised view of the world that has the affluent West reaping the just deserts of its greed, overconsuming itself to death.

Nonetheless, from about 1980 onwards this partial, selective, image-ridden thesis of an epidemic of diet-related killer diseases has become the medical consensus, and its doom-laden message impressed on the public with increasing vigour and certainty. The question is: why? One possibility is that those responsible for propagating the diet-disease thesis are themselves ignorant of the facts that contradict their arguments. In a way they could be forgiven, as the evidence in this chapter contradicting their assertions has either never been presented in this form before or has been 'lost' for a decade, that is, it can only be found by digging back deep into the medical literature and is not readily available in standard textbooks.

The second possibility is that those most closely involved in the thesis have deliberately misrepresented the strength of their case, and by selecting the facts that suit them, and ignoring others, have fabricated the case against the Western diet.

10

A Serious Deception

By the early 1980s the diet-heart thesis should have been in deep trouble. The trials set up to 'prove' that the disease could be influenced by changing diet, along with other aspects of people's lives, were about to produce their negative results; and the decline in heart disease in several countries had become so precipitate that it was becoming increasingly untenable to explain it away in terms of changing dietary patterns. But it was nonetheless from this time onwards that the British public was to become the victim of an almost continuous stream of warnings about the lethal nature of its food, reinforced by admonitions to adopt a better, 'healthier' diet.

Although it is difficult to prove there was a conspiracy to mislead, there were certainly many professional reputations on the line and two related developments indicate that the protagonists of the thesis were less than straightforward in the presentation of their case. Firstly, during this period the results of the trials and the changing pattern of heart disease in the US were presented in such a way that the rest of the medical community would fail to grasp just how damaging they were to conventional thinking about the causes of heart disease. Secondly, the main protagonists busied themselves in 'expert' committees where, under the illusion of considering and weighing the evidence in favour of their theories, they were able to assert their validity by fiat.

It is necessary in considering what follows to remember that by 1980 most doctors believed that heart disease was a 'lifestyle' disease, the evidence for the implication of food coming from the unchallenged cross-cultural and migrant studies. So it was less important to convince people that this was indeed the case than to limit the damage to the credibility of the thesis. First, therefore, the results of the trials published between 1981 and 1984 had to be explained away.

The five tests, it will be recalled, had demonstrated various facts relevant to the diet-heart thesis. The two trials in men with normal cholesterols (MRFIT in the US and the WHO trial in five European countries) had shown that encouragement to change the diet did not reduce the incidence of heart disease. The Oslo and LRCCPPT trials in men with ̄markedly elevated cholesterols had shown that stringent dietary measures or drugs could reduce (albeit with some difficulty) the incidence of heart disease in this group back to that of the rest of the population. And finally, the Finnish study had failed to show any benefit from encouraging dietary changes on a community basis in the province of North Karelia compared to that of Kuopio.

On the face of it, the results of the MRFIT trial should have been a considerable blow to the credibility and wisdom of the medical profession. One hundred and fifty principal investigators drawn from thirty different medical centres in the US, including most of the leading protagonists of the thesis, along with teams of doctors, nurses, nutritionists and health educators, had spent ten years and 150 million dollars trying and failing to prove the thesis. Some explanation was needed. The report of the trial suggested three.[1]

The first possibility was that the trial had failed because the thesis was incorrect. The MRFIT report dismisses this option as being 'inconsistent with most published data' (i.e. the circumstantial evidence from the cross-cultural and migrant studies). It acknowledges that 'some controversy has existed for years as to the precise benefits' of reducing fat in the diet, but affirms nonetheless that 'most scientific opinion, including public health groups, have concluded that benefits do indeed exist'. No further consideration is given to this interpretation of the result.

The second option was that the trial *had* been successful, but that this was concealed in the final result because one aspect of the treatment – the drugs used in the treatment of hypertension – had adversely affected those in the intervention group, thus concealing a possible benefit. This explanation has subsequently been shown to be incorrect.[2]

The third option became the accepted verdict. In setting up the trial in the early 1970s, it had been predicted that a certain number could be expected to get heart disease, and that the benefit of 'risk factor intervention', including changes in diet, would be revealed in a lower incidence of heart disease in the intervention compared to the control group. This had not happened, but in both groups there had been less heart disease than originally anticipated. The rationalisation was that the control group had also changed its diet and other aspects of its lifestyle (although there was no evidence to prove this) sufficiently to reduce its subsequent incidence of heart disease. It was therefore not possible to demonstrate an advantage from intervention because both groups had 'benefited' from lifestyle changes.

In view of the enormous efforts that had to go into encouraging those in the intervention group to change their lives, this would seem an unlikely explanation. More importantly, however, both groups had one-third less heart disease than had originally been predicted, which was the same figure as the overall decline in heart disease in the US during the period of the study. As there is no reason why those in the trial should have been exempt from this general trend, the real answer must be that the MRFIT trial refuted the thesis because it failed to demonstrate any benefit from dietary changes over and above the generalised trend of heart disease throughout the country; that is, the test demonstrated a generalised decline in heart disease rates from those of ten years earlier, but completely failed to show any link between diet and disease.

Nonetheless, this explanation that both groups benefited from lifestyle changes became the accepted verdict on the trial; it could not be accepted as a valid test of the thesis because it no longer compared the results of intervention (changing the diet) against the controls (not changing the diet). The trial was thus discredited and its crucial role as a test of the thesis could be ignored.

The failure of the WHO trial in five European countries was more easily dealt with. This trial was the largest (it involved 40,000 men) and in many ways the most significant test of whether encouraging lifestyle changes could prevent heart disease. As such, its full results should have been made widely available. But instead they were published in an obscure medical journal with the claim that 'intervention can be beneficial'.[3] This conclusion was based on presenting the results in a table of baffling and almost uninterpretable complexity. But by working through the table and totting up the mortality rates from heart disease in each group, it is ultimately possible to find the real results. Like those of the MRFIT trial, these reveal that, far from intervention being beneficial, there was zero difference in heart disease rates between the intervention and control groups.

The results of the North Karelia project were misinterpreted in the same way as those of the MRFIT trial. The rate of heart disease had fallen and this was evidence of the benefit of the intervention. The fact that heart disease had declined in all other parts of the country as well, and that it was showing the same pattern in many other countries, was ignored. The decline in the neighbouring control province of Kuopio was adduced as evidence that 'both provinces had benefited', that the citizens of Kuopio had decided to join those of Karelia in making important changes in their diet. Needless to say, nobody produced any evidence to prove that this had actually happened.

The discrediting and 'suppression' of the results of MRFIT and the WHO trial can be appreciated all the more readily by examining the way in which the LRCCPPT trial was presented to the public.[4] Here at last was a 'successful' trial, some return for the vast investment, which, presented in the right way, would go a long way to overcome the embarrassment of the earlier failures.

Anticipating the results before they were published in the medical journals (and so could be scrutinised by the medical community), the trial organisers summoned a press conference in early January 1984. The director, Basil M. Rifkind, hailed the results as the first study to 'demonstrate conclusively that the risk of heart disease can be reduced by lowering the blood cholesterol'. The President of the American Heart Association described it as a 'landmark' whose results had been 'eagerly awaited'.[5] Admittedly the trial had been in men with very high cholesterols, but the advance publicity claimed the results were of general significance, 'that they could and should be extended' to everyone.

The response to the press conference was a flurry of articles in marked contrast to the lack of publicity surrounding the earlier trials. 'Sorry it's true, cholesterol really is a killer', wrote *Time* magazine, and *Newsweek* quoted one of the leading organisers describing it as a 'milestone study that has implications for the health of all Americans'.[6] *Time* magazine followed its initial story two months later, putting a doleful egg and bacon on the front cover with the heading, 'Cholesterol, and now the bad news . . .'. Heart disease is 'a slow death without a fever', ran the story inside.

Of course the results of the LRCCPPT trial were not applicable to the general population and the extrapolation – that because giving a drug to those with very high cholesterols one can reduce heart disease, everyone can benefit from a change of diet – was unjustified. The conveniently forgotten MRFIT and the WHO trials had shown that. Nonetheless, the case was argued on the basis of a very simple-minded analysis: if heart disease in those with very high cholesterols could be reduced by major changes in diet (or drugs) then small changes in diet would reduce heart disease in those with normal cholesterols. Most people with heart disease have normal cholesterols; therefore a strategy directed to the mass of the population would have a greater impact on the disease than merely focusing on the minority with very high cholesterols.[7] This 'mass intervention' strategy, as it is known, is obviously false. Firstly, small changes in diet do not influence the level of cholesterol in the blood (self-regulation sees to that). Secondly, and even if they did, it would be irrelevant because normal cholesterol levels do not predict the subsequent risk of heart disease.

The theory of mass prevention was severely criticised in 1983 by Professor Michael Oliver of Edinburgh University. Quoting Oliver Cromwell's address to the Church of Scotland in 1650: 'I beseech you in the bowels of Christ, think it possible you may be mistaken', he noted:

> This admonition might now be appropriately addressed to some of the epidemiologists and the many overenthusiastic health educators concerned with prevention of heart disease. . . . Those debating what action should be taken to prevent heart disease would do well to reflect that 'mass action' has not yet been shown to be of benefit, like the Scots divines they may be wrong, they have misled themselves with a superficially attractive argument. This view is often taken up by health educationists many of whom have little knowledge of the biology and natural history of atherosclerosis or heart disease although this does not deter them from preaching a calvinistic lifestyle for us all.[8]

Oliver's admonitions had little impact and the 'superficially attractive argument', along with the unjustified extrapolations from the LRCCPPT trial, got the diet-heart thesis through the difficult problem of the failure of the MRFIT and WHO trials.

Flush with the successful promotion of the results of the LRCCPPT trial, the organisers mounted another highly publicised event, a 'consensus conference' on the prevention of heart disease under the auspices of the US National Institute of Health at the end of 1984.[9] This brought together all those involved in studying heart disease to discuss the issues and produce a statement restating the conventional wisdom. The report of the conference reviewed all the one-sided circumstantial evidence in favour of the thesis – the cross-cultural and migrant studies; jumped the negative results of the MRFIT and WHO trials straight to the results of the LRCCPPT as evidence of the benefits of reducing cholesterol levels; and so by extrapolation called for radical dietary changes for everyone.

> After careful review of the genetic, epidemiological and clinical trial evidence . . . we are persuaded that the blood cholesterol levels of most Americans are undesirably high in large part because of a high intake of saturated fat. All Americans should be advised to adopt a diet that reduces total dietary fat intake from 40 per cent to 30 per cent of total calories.

Not everyone was happy about the conference. Professor Michael Oliver wrote again to the *Lancet*:

> Those who initiated the idea were either naive or determined to use the forum for special pleading . . . the panel of jurists for the conference was selected to include experts who would predictably say that all levels of blood cholesterol in the US were too high and should be lowered, and of course that is exactly what was said. Well-orchestrated so-called consensus conferences with the implicit intention of exerting psychological and political pressure should not be permitted too loud a voice, however powerful the protagonists might appear to be, and be recognised as special pleading and treated as such.[10]

And in the same issue Professor Ahrens of Rockefeller University noted:

> Since many unanswered questions remain about the role of diet in the prevention of heart disease, it is remarkable that the press in the US has set out to sell the message that the diet-heart question has been solved . . . with more than tacit support from many of the scientists involved in the LRCCPPT trial.

Criticising the conference's decision to extrapolate from the LRCCPPT trial as a basis for making recommendations to the public, he observed: 'It promises benefits without giving the evidence to back up that promise. I am discouraged by the imbalance between the importance of the issues at stake and the manner in which the consensus conference has considered them.'[11]

But the bandwagon rolled on. The beginning of 1985 saw the launch in the US of a massive 'National Cholesterol Education Campaign' funded by twenty health-oriented organisations, intended to encourage public concern about the 'cholesterol problem', and to reaffirm in the public mind the validity of the diet-heart thesis and the importance of everyone changing their diets.

However, there still remained a second problem for the diet-heart protagonists: that of explaining away the exponential decline in heart disease in the US and other countries. This has been tackled by emphasising the marked decline in incidence in the US and inferring that it is due to 'lifestyle changes' and particularly a 'healthier diet'. Their point is made more effectively by placing the US decline in heart disease against other countries such as the UK and Sweden where heart disease has not fallen (Fig. 10.1).[12] The argument then goes: heart disease is preventable because it has declined in the US, and the fact that it has not declined in other countries is evidence that those countries have not been taking seriously enough the healthy diet message.

It is a classic misuse of statistics to prove a point. A cursory evaluation of the graph obviously argues against this interpretation of events. Why, if the phenomenon is due to a decline in fat consumption, is the relevant data not shown on the graph? Why has it not been declining in health-conscious Sweden; why is the pattern of the disease so similar in the US and Australia? Nonetheless, the inference that the decline in the US was due to changes in diet sustained probably the most powerful of all the myths that surrounded the diet-heart thesis.

The misrepresentation of the results of the trials, bolstered by the simplistic idea of 'mass prevention' and the propagation of the mythical explanation for the decline in heart disease in the US, saved the diet-heart thesis and even strengthened it at the crucial time when it was most threatened. The enormous efforts to promote it convinced many doctors, and why should they not believe? The circumstantial evidence from the cross-cultural and migrant studies went unchallenged. The MRFIT and WHO trials were minimised and forgotten. The link between a high cholesterol and heart disease had been confirmed by the LRCCPPT trial, and for those convinced of the diet-heart thesis there was a clear temptation to believe that its lessons could be extrapolated to everybody. The decline in heart disease in the US was adduced as evidence that heart disease could be prevented by dietary changes. It was this version of events that found its way into the medical textbooks, thus becoming part of the official body of knowledge on heart disease.[13]

Is this slender base really the foundation of the contemporary

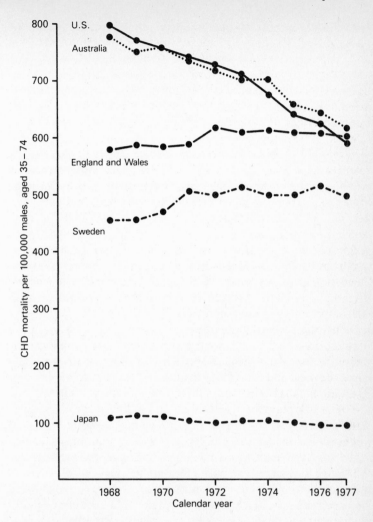

Fig.10.1 *Mortality rate from heart disease (CHD) in the U.S., Australia, England and Wales, Sweden and Japan 1968 – 1977*

orthodoxy? That it is is confirmed by examining the intellectual content of the expert committee reports produced between 1982 and 1987, each of which asserted unequivocally the urgency for changes in the Western diet. Each purported to examine the scientific evidence, although only one mentioned the trials and none critically examined the changing pattern of heart disease. They all came to the same conclusion: that the Western diet caused disease and needed to be changed radically.

A representative example – and perhaps the most important – was that from NACNE (National Advisory Committee on Nutrition Education).[14] It was published by the Health Education Council in 1983 under the chairmanship of Professor Philip James, who had been described in the press as 'being recognised as an outstanding member of the new generation of scientists and doctors who have studied the links between food and Western diseases'. The NACNE report was to become the bible of health educationists and others seeking to change the British diet. It claimed to be 'an authoritative statement of the present consensus over the whole field', which 'set out to rectify the relevant dietary defects of the population as a whole' on the theoretical basis of 'mass prevention' which 'opinion in the Western world was coming to favour as a prime basis for public health policy'. But its recommendations were based on false premises, misleading and selectively presented evidence, suppression of anything that might contradict its assertions and an uncritical avowal of contemporary opinion.

Thus, the section on heart disease in the report starts with the false premise, which if it were true would validate the diet-heart thesis but as it is not, invalidates it, that those who get heart disease eat more meat and dairy foods than those who do not. It argues that, applying the mass prevention theory, small reductions in fat intake for the whole population will have a greater effect on reducing heart disease than just treating those with high cholesterol levels: 'By reducing the fat intake of everybody by a modest amount, many more susceptible individuals will benefit despite the fact that their fat intake may have been only a little above average.'

In favour of this policy it cites two sources. Firstly, the authority of preceding expert committees: 'There is a striking degree of agreement among diverse expert committees in the Western world who have examined the issue that a marked reduction in saturated fat is indicated.' And secondly, the changing pattern of heart disease in the US: 'Compared with other Western countries Britain has a poor record in the prevention of heart disease, the rates in recent years only showing a slight decline compared with the US and Australia.' The report took no opportunity to discuss the actual results of the trials: they were just not mentioned.

In the next section on salt and blood pressure there is a similar eclectic approach to the evidence. The comparison between 'primitive' societies and Western countries appears to show that raised blood pressure (hypertension) is due to excess salt consumption, and one paper is quoted as apparently demonstrating the benefits of encouraging the public to reduce its salt intake. The reference here is: 'Abstracts of the 18th annual conference of cardiovascular epidemiology 1978, in the Cardiovascular Disease Newsletter no. 28'. Now, there are 2,000 to 3,000 papers published each year on hypertension, and the selection of this very obscure reference is intriguing. As Professor John Swales of Leicester University observed:

> Such a citation would not even get into the bibliography of hypertension. The use of such a publication to support a major recommendation is not acceptable scientific practice. When one recalls that it is the only study cited which actually purports to assess the consequences of carrying out a manoeuvre being recommended for the whole population for the next five years, it is fairly apparent that an enormous superstructure is being built on extremely weak foundations.[15]

Other papers in widely circulated medical journals which failed to show any benefit from salt reduction are not mentioned in the report. This partial interpretation of the evidence provoked all the leading scientists in the field of hypertension to write to the *Lancet* in complaint: the NACNE report, they said, had ignored the 'usual scientific methods for weighing evidence and giving advice'. It was instead indulging 'in an evangelical crusade to present a simplistic view of the evidence which will prove attractive to the media'.[16]

There is nothing unique about Professor James's optimistic selection of scientific 'facts', although the degree to which his report practised it is, perhaps, exceptional. It is certainly the more reprehensible because of the purpose for which it was intended. Scientific articles and reports in the medical press which practise selective (or dubious) interpretation of the facts will be picked up and criticised by those knowledgeable in the issues. The NACNE report was different in that it was to form the basis for the implementation of a social policy that would affect many people's lives, and would be promoted by others possibly unversed in the subtle details of the relationship between food and disease – health educators, policy makers and journalists. With this heavy and serious responsibility a balanced review of the evidence was vital. Rather the NACNE report dressed its opinions up in the garments of scientific objectivity, and in a tone of rationality that was utterly deceptive.

So it was on 'extremely weak foundations' that the NACNE report recommended widespread changes in the British diet, which became the litany of the health education movement in the following years. The dietary advice of the 1930s was now turned on its head as the promotion of the 'low-fat/high-fibre' diet became the panacea for the nation's ills. Boyd Orr had argued the need to increase the proportion of fat-based dairy foods rather than high-fibre foods such as bread and potatoes in the working-class diet, as a means of overcoming widespread malnourishment. Fifty years later the anathematised working-class diet was now the new 'healthy diet'. The advice to reduce fat consumption required abjuring cream, substituting skimmed milk for full milk and margarine for butter, cutting down on eggs and cheeses (like Stilton, Cheddar and Camembert), on full-fat yoghurt, processed meats, chocolate, cakes, biscuits and puddings, as well as reducing consumption of red meat by about one-third. The proscription on salt discouraged bacon, gammon, salt beef and mackerel, as well as its use in cooking. The admonishments on sugar discouraged sweets, soft drinks, biscuits and cakes, and extended to honey and syrups. To make up for abstaining from all these foods required increasing the intake of prodigious amounts of high-fibre foods, particularly bread and vegetables.

These changes in diet were a necessary consequence of the recommendation to reduce fat in the diet as meat and dairy foods are its most important source. However, the main thrust of the propaganda rapidly turned to focus specifically on those 'junk' foods – hamburgers, fish and chips, crisps and sweets – which were better able to sustain the imagery necessary to suggest that food might be injurious to health.

The publication of the NACNE report in 1983 signalled the beginning of a powerful and consistent campaign to convince the public. It rapidly became the 'official' document of the Health Education Council which then deployed its considerable resources to promote it. Once it had the approval of the HEC, it then became the standard text for all those involved in 'health promotion' who took the message into classrooms, village halls and lecture theatres across the nation. And those responsible for the provision of food in all manner of institutions, schools, hospitals and prisons started inflicting its recommendations on their captive audiences.

But most of all it allowed the HEC to approach television companies to launch major prime-time series of programmes based on the report. These ran alongside a blitzkrieg of similar programmes so that for a time it seemed there was nothing else on the television other than concerned health professionals informing the nation of the folly of its ways. Together they presented a non-contentious view of the scientific facts, expounded uniquely by those who believed in the diet-disease thesis with no dissension. Replete with images of food and death, they exploited the visual imagery to which the thesis lends itself so readily, elaborating on the traditional prejudice against 'convenience' or 'junk' foods to emphasise the heart-stopping properties of chips, the cancer-inducing properties of a meat pie.

The programmes first set the problem in general context:

> Our taste for unhealthy foods causes many of our health problems and the diseases that kill us . . . by making simple changes in what we eat, we can make dramatic changes to our health. (Commentator, *BBC Food and Health Campaign*)

And how were these discoveries made?

> It really turned out to be quite simple, all we had to do was look at the major national and international reports and they all came out with the same general message. (Philip James)

But might there not be some dissent?

> The major comment I would make is that most of those who are critical have no knowledge of the subject whatsoever . . . . and secondly many of them are self-serving. (Ancel Keys)

What about heart disease?

> The modern British diet is killing people in their thousands from heart attacks and it is because we eat far too much saturated fat. . . . I believe we know enough now to reduce the massive toll of heart attacks and strokes if we were to eat better. (Geoffrey Rose)

And cancer?

> Increasingly scientists are convinced that what we eat is as important as what we smoke in causing cancer. (Michael O'Donnell)

And salt?

> We strongly suspect that salt is important in causing raised blood
> pressure . . . if one looks at whole numbers of communities we
> find a very good relation between the amount of salt in the diet
> and the number of people with hypertension. (Colin MacGregor)

It would have been enough for the vigorous activities of health
educationists with the willing if unsophisticated connivance of the
media to persuade the public of the validity of the diet-disease
thesis. But the task was enormously strengthened by the activities of
the food industry, sections of which saw in the healthy diet message
a useful means of acquiring a larger section of the market.

The 'health food industry' benefited considerably from the new
concern about healthy foods and used the NACNE report's authority to promote its wares. The bread manufacturers sought and
obtained from the Health Education Council an official endorsement of their now approved 'high-fibre' product. The straight fight
for that limited section of the market, whether to spread butter or
margarine on the now endorsed bread, generated large-budget
advertising campaigns. The development of new products to fit in
with the new perceptions produced 'low-fat' yoghurts and soups
'with no added salt'. And then the big supermarket chains such as
Tesco and Sainsbury launched campaigns that suggested they took
the 'healthy eating' message seriously. As each of these initiatives
relied on massive advertising, they were in turn promoting the
diet-disease thesis. Wheeling the supermarket trolley through piles
of food labelled 'low-fat', or 'no added salt' was a none-too-subtle
reinforcement of the message.

There were subtler methods as well. The battle between the
butter and margarine industries stretches back through the century.
From the 1930s to the 1960s the tide had flowed with the dairy
industry, margarine trailing as an unsatisfactory substitute, a nutritionally less perfect product consumed by the working classes. The
stigma that associated margarine with relative poverty was difficult
to eradicate and in the post-war years its promotion rested on the
double assertion that it tasted the same as butter ('Honestly can't
tell the difference') and that it could be 'spread straight from the
fridge'. These rather unglamorous claims were transformed in the
1980s when margarine became a health product, a remedy against
heart disease.

It was Unilever that most effectively seized the opportunity with its Flora margarine. Although this contained as much fat as butter, it was 'high in polyunsaturates' – the 'good' fats which, taken in abundance in place of animal fats, can lower the level of blood cholesterol. Its manufacturers appreciated that the sales of this product would rise to the extent that the diet-heart thesis was generally accepted, and to this end set up the Flora Heart Disease Prevention project which sought to help health and other medical journalists to a better understanding of how fats cause heart disease by promoting a series of expensive trips around the world. These lucky beneficiaries travelled to a conference in Berlin (preceded by a few days sailing down the Rhine) to hear that the diet-heart thesis had been proved 'beyond reasonable doubt'; to Karelia in Finland to discover how a community-based heart disease prevention pro-gramme had reduced the rates of heart disease; to a conference in Florida to hear Basil Rifkind explain how the LRCCPPT trial was 'a landmark study with implications for the health of all Americans'.

As these trips were only providing evidence for the conventional wisdom of the time, there could be no suggestion that the opinions of this section of the media were being bought; but it was inspired marketing on the part of Unilever to realise that if medical and health journalists subscribed to the diet-heart thesis, it was a source of endless copy that would incidentally promote their product.

The appearance in the spring of 1985 of a series of articles in the national press on disease patterns in Japan indicated another successful Flora trip. The journalists on this trip were addressed by a Japanese scientist who argued that the Westernisation of the Japanese diet since the war years had brought in its wake a plague of Western killer diseases. He illustrated his point with a graph that showed a rise in the absolute number of deaths from heart disease over the period. Even by the standards of the diet-disease thesis this was a classic misuse of statistics. Firstly, the population of Japan had risen. Secondly, life expectancy had increased markedly to the longest in the world (evidence of the benefit of Westernising the diet?), so many more death certificates in Japan carried the patho-logically indeterminate diagnosis of 'heart disease' as a cause of death from 'old age'. And, as we have already seen, the death rate during this period from heart disease among middle-aged men, which the diet-heart thesis was meant to explain, had merely remained steady.[17]

Nonetheless, the notion that the Japanese were 'suffering' as a result of increasing Westernisation of the diet joined the attribution of the US decline in heart disease to a healthy diet as one of the more

powerful and resilient myths of the thesis. The most crucial point
was overlooked. During the period of 'Westernisation' of the diet
Japan had become the country with the longest-lived population in
the world, overtaking that of Sweden. If it is possible that such
essentially disparate societies as Japan and Sweden could each
ensure a long and useful life for its citizens, how could food be a
cause of 'epidemics of disease' (Fig. 10.2)?

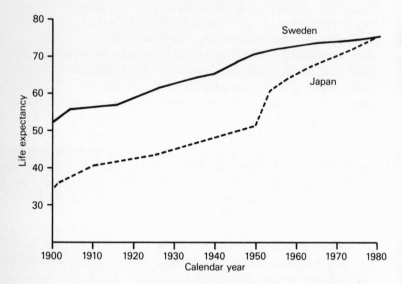

Fig.10.2 *Japan and Sweden have the longest life expectancy in the
world even though their dietary patterns are very different*

It was not the function of the Flora Heart Disease Prevention
Project to evaluate or interpret these misleading statistics, merely to
set up the situation in which they could be noted down and rewritten
as further evidence for the validity of the thesis that had done so well
by their product.

Against the sophistication of Unilever's Flora operation, its
competitor, the Butter Information Council, made a poor showing.
Given the current of the time, it is difficult to see how it could have
been otherwise. The only reward for the Council's pains in support-
ing a conference in London that took a sceptical look at the thesis
was a *Sunday Times* story – 'Angry doctors lash butter industry on
heart disease' – quoting Professor Geoffrey Rose: 'The high intake
of fat including butter in the British diet is the main single reason
why there is so much heart disease.'

The final accolade for the thesis was its incorporation into the manifestos of the political parties. One of the great advantages of the diet-disease thesis, which in part explains its wide currency, is that its message can be interpreted as favouring both ends of the political spectrum. For the Left, the problem was that people were dying from preventable diseases because reputedly they could not afford to buy the now-approved healthy foods. For the Right, the suggestion was that people should be more responsible for their own health, and if only they consumed a better diet the state would not have to spend so much money on running the health service.

In 1985 the Labour Party produced a research document written by Professor James (of NACNE fame) on the relationship between food and disease. It formed the basis for their 'Charter for Prevention': 'The UK leads the world league tables for heart disease which is directly related to unhealthy diet', it said, and proposed the development of dietary goals which would be publicised widely with 'effective nutrition campaigns' mounted around them. The following year the Junior Minister of Health chastised the irresponsible northerners on their fondness for chips. With the run-up to the General Election of 1987, the Government launched a lavish health education programme based on the assertions of the diet-heart thesis (*Look after Your Heart*). It emphasised the individual's responsibility for preventing the disease by making the correct dietary changes, and incidentally deflected public concern from the more pressing political problems of the health service.

By 1986 the protagonists of the diet-disease thesis could feel well satisfied. Their beliefs were now fully incorporated into the medical textbooks and public policy, and engraved on the consciousness of the public. And yet none of it is actually true; a vast edifice of belief has been built on shaky foundations and is sustained only by careful management of the winds that threatened it.

So why is it that a traditionally sceptical and phlegmatic profession like that of medicine could have been persuaded? Or, to put it another way: what are the problems in contemporary medicine that have allowed it to flourish?

11
Absurdity Flourishes

The simplest and most powerful argument against the diet-heart thesis is neither the flawed nature of the circumstantial evidence in its favour, nor that it has been refuted by experiment; but that it is an outrage against common sense.

Man is uniquely capable of adapting to a vast variety of different patterns of food intake, and in the latter part of the twentieth century – for the first time in recorded history – his average life span approximates to that of the biological life span. Yet when it comes to explaining the commonest cause of premature death in males, a novel disease that has been rising and falling exponentially over the last several decades, the reason given is that it is due to the type of food its victims eat. There is no analogy in the whole corpus of medical knowledge to suggest that food can be lethal in this way. Even so, this explanation is for the most part accepted uncritically, even though it is not possible to show that those dying from the disease in any one country eat more fat than anyone else, or that the marked rise and fall of the disease is paralleled by changes in the pattern of fat consumption.

What is remarkable is that this thesis should have currency at a time when medicine has reached an almost unimaginable level of refinement in other fields. To understand how absurdity has flourished in the midst of intellectual sophistication requires a closer examination of the curious history of post-war medicine.

It is a common assumption that medicine operates on an upward curve of knowledge, that the application of science to the study of disease brings each year new insights and new understandings. The reality of the history of medicine in the period since the last war is very different. For twenty-five years, from 1945 till about 1970, medicine experienced one of those revolutionary convulsions that punctuate the history of human achievement. In an astonishingly short period of time, and in each and every medical speciality, what was inconceivable only a few years previously became commonplace. Tuberculosis had virtually been eliminated and was anyhow eminently curable, and the life-threatening childhood infections of diphtheria and polio had been eradicated. It was possible to repair the most complex developmental abnormalities of the heart in the first month of life. New treatments could powerfully influence serious illnesses previously virtually untreatable – schizophrenia, epilepsy, asthma and dozens of others. They could even cure some cases of childhood cancer. Hips, hearts and kidneys could be replaced, pacemakers inserted, arteries plumbed. And then in the 1970s this convulsion of innovation subsided as if medicine had reached some ceiling of theoretical and practical achievement. New treatments were still being introduced but at a fraction of their previous rate.

So post-war medicine can be divided into two phases: a golden epoch of twenty-five years of almost continuous achievement, followed by a fallow period of fifteen years that is with us still. In this the experience of medicine is no different from that of any other scientific discipline; all are characterised by spurts of growth followed by years of quiescence. Perhaps 1945 is an arbitrary moment to pinpoint the beginnings of this golden epoch as the foundations for much of the success of the following years had already been well laid in the application of the scientific method to the problems of illness. But around that moment two phenomena coalesced with remarkable potency.

The first was the 'knock-on' effect in which several distinct discoveries came together at one moment to form the basis of further progress. A good example of the way this effect works is the 'ultimate' operation of heart transplantation. The first transplant in 1968 might have seemed to be a shot in the dark, but it was in fact built on a long tradition of increasingly sophisticated cardiac surgery, and on developments in many different disciplines, particularly pharmacology and anaesthetics. In a sense, they were all leading to the transplant.

Thus, in the late 1940s developments in blood transfusion and the introduction of powerful new anaesthetics encouraged surgeons to consider relatively straightforward operations on the heart – the repair of simple congenital defects and of damaged heart valves. The early 1950s saw the introduction of new drugs to control abnormal rhythms of the heart; and in 1956 came the first heart-lung machine, which allowed the function of the heart to be 'bypassed' temporarily, by siphoning the blood outside the body to be oxygenated and then returned to the circulation. Now the chest could be opened, the heart stopped and much more sophisticated surgery performed on it. There remained the most difficult problem in transplanting organs: overcoming the desire on the part of the body's immune system to reject foreign tissue. But this had been made possible by the discovery of two groups of 'immunosuppressant' drugs – the steroids in the late 1940s and azathioprine in 1952. With these and other impediments to the operation already resolved, it only required the courage to apply them for the first time. In the operation, all the developments that made it possible came together to produce a 'knock-on' effect: a daring advance in surgical practice.

None of this would have been possible if it had not been for the second main agent behind the golden epoch of medicine: the 'accidental' discovery of a vast range of useful drugs. This process had started with the discovery of sulphonamide antibiotics in 1936, as part of a routine screening programme for antibacterial chemicals, and of penicillin in 1940, based on Fleming's chance observations of a decade earlier. Both finds were made without direct reference to the specific nature of the diseases which they were destined to treat; that is, it was not necessary to understand the pathology of the infectious diseases to find an empirical treatment for them. Rather than spending years trying to understand the causes and mechanisms of illnesses (if indeed they were understandable) it seemed necessary only to 'screen' chemical compounds by administering them to laboratory animals to see whether they had an interesting effect that might have some exploitable therapeutic value. During the post-war years literally millions of compounds were screened in this way, producing most of the drugs in common use today. The process was not completely blind. Past experience of the effects of chemical compounds were reinvestigated; chance or serendipity played an important role when the introduction of a drug for one condition revealed useful side effects that could be used to treat other quite separate illnesses. And there were a few drugs that were designed to fulfil a specific purpose. But for the most part, like the gold prospectors of old, the pharmaceutical companies ran to and fro, stumbling every so often on nuggets of gold sticking above the ground.

There is obviously a limit to the knock-on effect of developments in medicine and the accidental discovery of drugs. By the time it is possible to transplant hearts, there is little more to be achieved in the field of cardiac surgery. After screening millions of compounds for their potential therapeutic activity, the barrel becomes a bit spare; and although theoretically there might still be a few unexpected revelations, few have come to light in recent years. This, then, was the point reached by the early 1970s. Despite increasingly vast funds allocated to medical research and invested by the pharmaceutical companies, the return in terms of useful innovations was patchy indeed and in marked contrast to the preceding twenty-five years. True, there were new 'growth areas' in the application of genetic science, and there was much to be gained by defining more accurately the role of many of the drugs introduced with such abandon earlier; but the major breakthroughs to which medicine had become so accustomed were few. As of 1986, the vast majority of drugs in common use had been discovered before 1970.

As time has passed it has become possible to assess what was achieved during the golden epoch. Although the whole range of medicine had benefited, the actual understanding of the mechanisms and causes of disease had changed little. There were, of course, exceptions: smoking had been incriminated in lung diseases, some new viruses had been found to cause specific diseases such as hepatitis, glandular fever, Burkitt's lymphoma and, most recently, AIDS. But the vast bulk of diseases remained as obscure as ever, whether they were the illnesses contracted at any period of life – diabetes, rheumatoid arthritis, multiple sclerosis – or the diseases of ageing – circulatory disorders and cancer. Likewise, some previously incurable conditions were now curable: bacterial infectious diseases had fallen to the all-conquering antibiotics; previously fatal surgical defects of the heart and ruptured aneurysms could be repaired; infertility could be treated with drugs or surgery. But it remained the case that the much larger contribution of this period had been in controlling the symptoms of the chronic diseases, and mitigating the effects of the diseases of ageing.

The discoveries of the time were real enough, but their source was the application of empirically acquired knowledge rather than an insight into the complex biological problems of disease. This engendered the illusion that medicine understood more than it really did, that it could provide answers to all problems. Seen in this light, it is possible to appreciate the full implausibility of the diet-disease thesis, the gross discrepancy between its claims to understanding and the actual state of medical knowledge. The number of diseases for which a specific cause had been identified were very few, yet here the assertion was being made that not one but many complex illnesses could be prevented by simple changes in diet. But the thesis was very much a child of its time. Hatched in the 1960s when the progress of medicine was at its most dramatic, its claim that heart disease was preventable might have appeared only too plausible to its originators and could scarcely be contested if so many other promises of medicine were being fulfilled. The notion that science might remain profoundly ignorant about the causes of almost all diseases was not widely held.

Rather, the practical achievements of the golden epoch were such as to encourage a belief in the wisdom and effectiveness of medicine, and to help governments and the public accept the explanations of the medical profession. The escalating rise in premature heart disease desperately required just such an explanation and, with the diet-heart thesis, the public got both an explanation and a solution. In the absence of contending theories it filled a vacuum of knowledge and gave heart disease an identity, defining it in such a way that it lost its terror. It was better to know that the disease was caused by saturated fats than to admit that its cause was not known. And if the diet-heart thesis was widely accepted, who was to doubt the general validity of the wider diet-disease thesis?

In addition, no government or public-spirited body could fail to be impressed by the breathtaking progress of the early post-war years and this generated a faith (shared by many doctors) in medicine's endless possibilities. If there was not a ready answer it only meant not enough money had been spent in finding one. A paucity of funds rather than a paucity of ideas was seen as the only brake on progress. The medical establishment prospered with vastly expanded numbers, new hospitals and research institutions; and the funds to investigate the diet-heart thesis were readily available, running in the end into hundreds of millions of pounds.

By the time the major trials of the thesis were started in the early 1970s, the golden epoch was beginning to fade – but there was no way of knowing that at the time. So, flush with optimism, they were launched. They never should have been, as even a moderately sceptical examination of the evidence from the cross-cultural and migrant studies would have been sufficient to suggest they were unlikely to produce the expected results. But they were, and when ten years later they failed to prove anything other than what was in a sense predictable (that it was possible to reduce the risk of heart disease in those with very high cholesterols), there should have been a lot of explaining to do.

The trouble, however, with very expensive theories is that it becomes increasingly difficult to accept they are wrong. It was too much to ask those protagonists who had invested such vast research funds and their own professional lives to say, 'We're sorry, it seems as if we have made a mistake. We were full of optimism that heart disease could be prevented by dietary change, but now it seems we were wrong.' Instead it appears that, consciously or not, they set out to convince the rest of the profession and the public of the validity of the thesis by a process of selection and suppression of the relevant evidence.

The credibility of the diet-heart thesis thus rested on several planks. There was the widespread belief in the wisdom of medicine generated by the success of the post-war years; an illusion, shared as much by doctors as by the public, that medicine understood more than it really did. There was the personal commitment of those most closely identified with the thesis, whose profound comments on the role of diet in disease provided the authoritative assertions it so badly needed. But its widespread acceptance was also enormously strengthened by a paradoxical reaction to the very success of the golden epoch. The increasingly technological orientation of medicine had begun to evoke for the public the chilling spectre of illness now placing them in the hands of white-coated technicians in vast palaces of disease employing powerful drugs with uncertain side effects. The diet-heart thesis was there to say this fate could be avoided if individuals 'took health into their own hands'. If change in diet was going to prevent heart disease and cancer, it was a treatment that seemed not only sensible but eminently preferable to that of being an alienated patient in a lonely hospital bed.

This same reaction is seen in the simultaneous rise in the popularity of 'alternative' medicine, with which the diet-heart thesis has so much in common. Both emerged from a disappointment at the failure of medicine to achieve certain specific ends, whether it be the prevention of heart disease or the cure of some chronic condition that had eluded the ministrations of orthodox treatment; and so both were indebted to the success of post-war medicine in generating expectations that could only be disappointed. But both also relied on a reaction to technological solutions in favour of more personal ones, and both made unevaluated claims of therapeutic success. The diet-disease thesis and alternative medicine thus entered into a symbiotic relationship. Alternative medicine gained acceptance by the apparent authority of scientific medicine's pronouncements on the simple dietary solutions to disease; the diet-disease thesis gained credence from the widespread simplistic anti-scientific ideology that alternative medicine promoted.

Irrespective of all the explanations as to why the diet-disease thesis prospered when it did, it never could have done so without the active connivance of its protagonists. For many the motivation must remain opaque. For some, there are more obvious attractions. There is much money to be made from making people anxious about their cholesterol levels. Measuring the amount of cholesterol in the blood cost worried private patients in the US an estimated 100 million dollars in 1985; and there are rich rewards from the promotion of cholesterol-lowering drugs. But more interesting than the motives of individuals and companies is another question: why has the discipline of epidemiology become so compromised in promoting the thesis?

Epidemiology sets itself the twin tasks of correlating by statistical methods diseases with possible causes in the environment, and then, by applying the logic of statistics (as illustrated by Bradford Hill's canons of proof), of determining whether the correlation is truly causal. The legacy of this method of investigation is enormously impressive. It revealed the contagious nature of cholera before the cause of cholera was discovered; it pointed to the vitamin deficiency syndromes long before the chemical structure of vitamins was revealed; it proved beyond all doubt the relationship between smoking and lung cancer. And in each case the results of applying that knowledge are immediate and striking. Legislate for clean water and cholera disappears. Improve the diet and beriberi is eliminated. If the public were to stop smoking, lung cancer would virtually disappear. This is medicine on a grand scale: the institution of simple preventive measures which have an impact on disease much greater than the often seemingly futile activities of their colleagues in white coats with their potent remedies.

And yet looking at the diet-disease thesis is like being in a hall of mirrors: nothing is as it appears. Statistics, when correctly deployed, not only accurately reflect reality but are capable of profound insights into the natural world, giving coherence to apparently disconnected phenomena. But in this case reality has become distorted: the fact that most people in the Western world live out their natural lifespan has been turned around to throw back the reflection of a vast burden of disease and disability caused by the

food we eat. Epidemiology seems to have travestied its best tradi-
tions: why has this happened?

As the health of the Western nations improved, so the opportunities declined for the striking and effective insights into the nature of
disease and methods of prevention that characterised the early
history of epidemiology. And in the immediate post-war years,
when the emphasis was so heavily oriented towards the application
of empirically acquired knowledge, it began to appear as if
epidemiology's contribution to medicine was becoming increasingly
diminished. The demonstration of the causative relationship between smoking and lung cancer could have been its last great fling –
until the arrival of the diet-heart thesis. Here again was the old
tradition of epidemiology rediscovered. Once again it appeared that
the application of statistical methods had found in the environment
both the cause of an important disease and its solution.

The temptation to run with this theory was considerable. Its
protagonists were defence, prosecution, judge and jury of their own
theories. Unlike the practice of medicine, where new discoveries
are applied by many and discarded if found to be ineffective,
there was no independent judge of the diet-disease thesis because
those promoting it were in a position to ensure that the evidence
disproving it was kept out of the realms of public knowledge.

The natural world is, however, a hard taskmaster. It does not
readjust to fit in with the way fallible scientists believe it should
behave, and ultimately the inconsistencies of erroneous theories
become insupportable. Then it becomes imperative to place incorrect theories in the best possible light, to suggest they are of general
or universal significance, to defend them by throwing up a stockade
of scientific obscurantism and authority. What other interpretation
can explain why the cross-cultural studies were used to support the
thesis even though comparisons between countries do not hold for
such an obvious cause and effect as smoking and lung cancer? How
else to explain why the Japanese migrant studies were produced as
evidence of the role of diet in heart disease when even a cursorily
sceptical review of the evidence throws up the experience of the
Swedish migrants to refute the inference; or why it was asserted that
the decline in heart disease in the US was due to dietary changes
when no changes of sufficient magnitude had taken place? In brief,
what else can explain the perpetuation of a fundamental confusion
between association and causality when that crucial distinction is at
the very centre of the discipline itself?

12
Final Meditations

For every problem there is a solution, neat, plausible and wrong.
(H. L. Mencken)

We have followed the rise and fall of contradictory but neat and plausible explanations of disease, with their equally contradictory but neat and plausible solutions: how in the 1930s widespread malnourishment was only resolvable by a marked increase in the consumption of meat and dairy products, and how in the 1980s an 'epidemic' of diet-related diseases of affluence could only be prevented by a major reduction in exactly the same foods.

Although the nutritional wisdoms are contradictory, they have so much in common they could be different sides of the same coin.

The circumstances in which they arose are very similar. Both wisdoms were preceded by genuine and important scientific observations on which they relied to sustain their credibility by analogy. The 1930s' wisdom followed the fascinating discoveries of the role of vitamins in health, particularly the role of vitamin D in preventing rickets. If vitamin D-rich dairy foods prevented rickets, they should also promote growth; and if rapid early growth was equated with health, then a high consumption of dairy foods was 'healthy'. The 1980s' version inherited the confirmation of the role of smoking in lung cancer. If a very common and lethal disease was caused by a social habit such as smoking, it was possible that other common diseases were also caused by other social habits such as diet. If lung cancer could be prevented by stopping smoking, changing the diet could prevent heart disease.

Both wisdoms filled a vacuum of achievement, becoming popular at a time when there was a sense of the medicine's limited ability to influence disease. By the 1930s the scientific tradition in medicine had been flourishing for over fifty years and in the germ theory of disease had revealed most of the bacteria that cause infectious disease. Yet despite this knowledge, the ability to cure these illnesses remained frustratingly small. Nutrition stepped in as an all-embracing method for improving the health of the nation. In the 1980s nutritional explanations of disease again became prominent when the therapeutic revolution of the post-war years had become exhausted, and there was a growing realisation that those therapeutic discoveries could do much less to influence disease than had previously been thought. The diet-disease thesis proposed a messianic answer to these problems.

Both involved, too, a false characterisation of the medical problem they intended to solve. In the 1930s it was suggested there was widespread malnourishment because whole classes failed to achieve arbitrarily defined Recommended Daily Allowances of certain nutrients. In the 1980s diseases powerfully determined by ageing (and so prevalent in societies where the natural lifespan began to approximate to the biological lifespan) were said to be caused by the diet of affluence. Both sought evidence for these claims not by a study of the problems themselves, but from elsewhere. Nobody demonstrated widespread malnourishment; only that there was a height differential between the social classes. Nobody showed that those who suffered from heart disease had different diets from anyone else; only that cross-cultural and migrant studies revealed differing patterns of disease in different countries.

Both also relied on the extrapolation from scientific observations about highly particular groups of people to infer that those observations were of universal significance. In the 1930s it was possible that relatively impoverished diets might be improved by the addition of dairy food supplements or other sources of calories; and in the 1980s that those with very high levels of cholesterol in the blood might reduce their risk of heart disease by radically reducing their consumption of fat.

Both sets of nutritional solutions, when submitted to the rigorous test of scientific experiment, were not vindicated; and in both cases the results of those experiments were minimised or ignored. Unable to find vindication within the scientific domain, both were nonetheless sold to the public by similar means.

Both invoked a semantic description of meat and dairy foods that powerfully prejudged the conclusion they intended to draw. First they were 'protective foods'; later they came under the sinister title of 'saturated fat'. Both invoked powerful imagery of the role of food in health to sustain the suggested mechanisms of disease. First there was a relative lack of 'flesh- and bone-forming' dairy foods in the diets of the working class to explain a presumed state of poor physique and ill health. Then in the 1980s fat furred up arteries, salt overloaded the circulation, and heavy, loose stools from a high-fibre diet cleansed the bowel of presumed cancer-forming agents.

And finally, both bypassed the inconvenient paucity of experimental evidence by relying on the pronouncements of specially selected 'expert' committees to assert their validity by fiat.

The contradictory nutritional wisdoms do appear as two sides of the same coin and that coin is the Western diet. The distinguishing feature of this diet is that it is relatively high in meat and dairy foods – or 'saturated fat'. For those who seek a link between food and disease that means there are two available permutations. Either there is too little of these foods in the diet and health will be improved by increasing them, as was suggested in the 1930s; or there is too much and health will be improved by decreasing them, as suggested in the 1980s. The similarities arise from the circumstances within which, and the methods by which, science has been deployed to substantiate one or other position. That much is clear.

But it still leaves unanswered the question of why these scientific versions of reality have become incorporated into the public consciousness to form the two contradictory versions of what constitutes 'healthy' eating – more meat and dairy products in the 1930s, less in the 1980s. It is obviously unlikely that these healthy diets became popular because the public was impressed by the subtlety of the scientific arguments; rather, it is more probable that the contradictions touch and exploit much deeper polarities of perception – political, philosophical, religious and sexual – within society. At its simplest, the 1930s' endorsement of meat and dairy foods exploits those perceptions which emphasise 'high church' virtues of sensuousness and élitism; the 1980s' rejection of those same foods exploits opposing perceptions which emphasise instead 'low church' virtues of asceticism and egalitarianism.

To elaborate: all complex societies are hierarchically structured, and people's sense of their position in that hierarchical pile is reinforced by a multitude of subtle and not so subtle distinctions – the size and style of their homes, how they speak, how many servants they have, how fast their horses run and so on. One particularly powerful and expressive distinction is the pattern of food consumption. An élite with the money to buy expensive foods, the leisure to explore the infinite culinary resources of the natural world and the opportunity to employ others to do the hard work in the kitchen, will view food not just as a means of supplying calories but as a cultural activity and a source of sensuous pleasure. For those less privileged, the bounty of the aristocrat's table might be a source of resentment; or they might make a virtue of necessity and emphasise the virtues of the simple life, of an uncomplicated attitude to food.

Patterns of food consumption predict attitudes to food, and in this context can be seen to reflect traditional conflicts between groups or classes within society: 'There's fat meat in your kitchen and there are well-fed horses in your stable, yet the people look hungry and in the outskirts of the city men drop dead from starvation.'[1] In more recent times, a new twist to this old paradigm is to be found in the reaction to the conspicuous consumption of the 'new' ruling class in Communist countries. Thus the Yugoslav patriot Djilas takes a dim view of this aspect of life in Stalin's Russia:

> We became inured to all sorts of things in the Soviet Union. As children of the Party and Revolution who had acquired faith in themselves and the faith of the people through ascetic purity, we could not help being shocked at the drinking party that was held for us on the eve of our departure to the front. . . . Girls who were too pretty and too extravagantly made up to be waitresses brought in vast quantities of the choicest victuals – caviar, smoked salmon and trout, fresh cucumbers and pickled aubergine, boiled hams, cold roast pigs, hot meat pies and piquant cheeses, borsch, sizzling steaks and finally cakes a foot thick and platters of fruit under which the tables began to sag.[2]

Attitudes towards 'sagging tables' might be important in the class conflict, but they also symbolise a philosophical divide between spiritual and material values. There are those who will look admiringly at John the Baptist and his exotically wholesome diet of locusts and wild honey, while others will join Athenaeus in his glorification of the joys of the material world:

> And then two slaves brought in a well rubb'd table
> And then another, and another, till
> The room was fill'd, and then the hanging lamps

> Beamed bright and shone upon the festive crowns,
> And herbs, and dishes of rich delicacies.
> And then all arts were put in requisition
> To furnish forth a most luxurious meal.[3]

This spiritual-materialist antithesis in people's attitude towards food is further strengthened by the close connection between food and the other major sensual activity of man – sex. Lévi-Strauss points out that cooking and sexual activity both centre upon the household, and as the same individuals are frequently involved, the cooking of food by the women can be seen as reciprocating the coital act of the male. The Cambridge anthropologist Jack Goody observes in addition that the word 'to eat' in certain African cultures is frequently used for sex, and covers much of the semantic field of the word 'enjoy' in English. Furthermore, the supposed virtues of sexual abstention are closely linked to ascetic attitudes towards food.[4] Goody cites Marco Polo's observation that 'the regular order of the Yogi carry abstemiousness to extremes'. Not only do they 'fast all the year round and never drink anything but water', but 'they go without a stitch of clothing and when asked why they display their private parts reply they are not ashamed since "we cannot do sin with them"'. Closer to our own culture, Rules 39 and 40 of the order of St Benedict parallel the Yogi's ascetic attitudes to both food and sex, for, along with the vow of celibacy, the consumption of animal flesh is forbidden except in cases of physical infirmity.

'Scientific' notions of what constitutes a healthy diet are thus immediately and profoundly validated by many pre-existing and predetermined polarities of belief. The question is why in Britain over the last fifty years did the élitist/sensuous extreme implicit in emphasising the virtues of a high-fat diet flourish in the 1930s, to be replaced by the egalitarian/ascetic low-fat diet of the 1980s?

The answer would seem to be that during these different periods the contending nutritional wisdoms embodied utopian aspirations, promises of solutions to what were at these different times perceived to be the major problems of society.

In broad terms, the most pressing problem in Britain in the 1930s was that of widespread poverty arising from unemployment. Boyd Orr gave this view a 'scientific' basis by providing evidence which purported to show that poverty brought with it widespread malnourishment: whole sections of society were enfeebled because they failed to achieve a predetermined goal of optimum nutrition. As this goal was based on a comparison of the food consumption patterns of the rich and poor, it led logically to the conclusion that optimum nutrition meant embracing the nutritional habits of the upper social classes, with a diet high in meat and dairy foods – a 'high-fat' diet.

The strong egalitarian sentiments of the time further promoted this wisdom. If the lot of the poor could be improved by a more equitable distribution of the fatty meats of the aristocrat's table, then the diet of the upper class should by rights become the diet of all. In the ideal world all would eat a lot of meat and dairy foods, all would be tall and healthy.

The contrary nutritional wisdom of the prosperous 1980s was based on the supposition that prosperity and affluence were in some way harmful. So when, for the first time in history, most people were nearly living out their natural lifespan, it was the diseases powerfully determined by ageing – cancer and disorders of the circulatory system – which became the diseases of civilisation, diseases caused by affluence. The utopian solution was to be found in emphasising the contrary virtues of asceticism, embracing a low-fat, high-fibre diet as a means of preventing those diseases.

So what does this mean? Firstly, it should be no surprise that the versions of a healthy diet are contradictory, because in broad terms the two ways in which food can be linked with illness in our society are themselves contradictory: either there is too little or too much saturated fat in the diet. Secondly, while the credibility of these versions of the healthy diet starts from the presentation of evidence purporting to show that people are either under- or overnourished, their strength is that the proffered solutions exploit much profounder political and philosophical polarities of belief in our society in a way that presents dietary change as the means of achieving a better world.

This, however, provides only the general context within which the different versions of the healthy diet appear plausible at different times. They are in the end believed by individuals because of the almost universal conviction that food can influence health.

It is everyone's experience that food can produce physical sensations both good and bad, whether it is a mediocre meal in a restaurant where the sensation of discomfort is compounded by the knowledge that it will have to be paid for, or a snack that is insufficient to satisfy hunger, or a Christmas lunch where the subsequent sense of overindulgence is compounded by feelings of guilt. It is easy to attribute to these sensations a greater significance than they really possess, reinforced by the rhetoric of popular nutrition in which ingredients are deemed good or bad depending on whether they are 'refined' or 'unrefined', 'natural' or 'convenience' foods.

'Refined foods' are the classic example. For centuries, refined white bread was considered superior to brown because it was believed that removing the useless germ by milling made flour more nutritious as well as more palatable and expensive. But if the argument is changed to suggest that something of nutritional value is instead lost in the process of milling, then refinement acquires the opposite connotations of enfeeblement and corruption.

Similarly, one of the great successes of the promotion of the current healthy diet is the way in which popular nutrition has transformed the scientific arguments against meat and dairy food into a more readily comprehensible approval of 'natural' as against 'convenience' foods. In the ideal world implied by this antithesis, everyone might perhaps go out in the morning, kill a boar, bring it home, dress it with wild herbs and eat it washed down by grapes from the vineyard. This is 'natural', healthy eating. The rise of urban civilization, however, has made this method of obtaining calories inconceivable for any but the most privileged; and so to allow the vast populations of cities access to a moderately varied diet, food has had to be processed – canned or frozen or (more recently) freeze-dried and irradiated. In short, it has had to be made more 'convenient' for the consumer. The ship's biscuit is as much a convenience food as a can of peas, yet (as with the unrefined/refined antithesis) the mere fact that it has been tampered with makes it in the eyes of some a nutritionally less wholesome product. It certainly might taste less good than the 'natural' article; but if the alternative is not to have access to these foods at all, that is simply a matter of palatability – as opposed to nutrition – we have to put up with.

Over the last few years the antipathy towards 'convenience' foods has become equated with the classic example of 'junk' food – the hamburger. Objectively it could be said that there is nothing wrong with the hamburger – a thick piece of meat providing lots of minerals and good quality animal protein, with a small vegetable garnish also providing a quota of vitamins, all encased in a brown bun high in the desirable fibre: nutritionally, a perfectly balanced meal. It may also contain a few chemicals, but nobody makes a hue and cry about the chemicals in the average apple skin.

In the world of popular nutrition, the hamburger does not have a chance. Dispersed in factory style outlets and despised by the middle class, its very popularity and ubiquity become proof enough that the Western diet is harmful. Now it might not be a good idea to eat only hamburgers, just as it might not be a good idea to eat only apples or carrots; but characterizing this type of food as 'junk' and associating it with grossness and ill-health proves a powerful incentive to opt for the current version of the healthy diet. Just, indeed, as an aversion to the presumed working-class diet of the 1930s – tea, bread and margarine – was an incentive to aspire to the healthier diet of more dairy products and meat.

With such a multiplicity of influences, conscious and unconscious, affecting public attitudes to the role of food in health, it is scarcely surprising that ideas about 'healthy eating' are so pervasive. As a counterbalance it makes it all the more important, therefore, to remember that 'there is no such thing as an ideal diet'.

The false remedies of nutritional 'science' in the 1930s vitiated a solution to the problems of the hungry in the post-war years, and led, through the uncritical avowal of vitamins, to a completely novel disease in the 1950s – idiopathic hypercalcaemia of infancy. Can it be said that the prevailing nutritional wisdoms are harmful in a similar way?

Under the guise of health education, the public has been taught to link pleasure with disability and death. In classrooms up and down the land children are told that the foods they enjoy – crisps, chocolate, sausages, fish and chips and hamburgers – can be lethal, while less popular foods are uniquely good for them – dried bananas, muesli, brown rice and so on.

It all sounds rather familiar. Pleasure is sinful, self-denial virtuous. But it is more than that. You did not know this particular pleasure was sinful, and now we are telling you; but luckily we can also tell you how to redeem your sin by following our guidelines on what you should eat. This is heady stuff for impressionable minds. Children are vulnerable to the imprint of their early instruction. When this involves religious beliefs some, on reaching adulthood, will find new and invariably better reasons for continuing them and some will shrug them off, but others will feel guilt, caught in the conflict between their desires and their early beliefs. If the religious analogy is appropriate, then a generation of children is now growing up which will instinctively regard the fish and chip shop as a haven of death, and some may well become unhealthily neurotic about food as a result.

The adult mind is less impressionable, but the sanctions held over adults to change their diet are more intense. By middle age the desire to live a long and useful life becomes a matter of some urgency. By this time too many will have familiarity with death and the authoritative media message that the British diet is 'probably the most atrocious in the world', that 'Britain is top of the league in the heart disease tables', that 30 per cent of cancers are caused by too much fat in the diet, will be intimately affecting. Foods previously esteemed in our culture will be seen as uniquely lethal, and many people will assume that adopting a less palatable, 'more wholesome' diet will reduce the risk of dying prematurely. Thus pleasure is denied and a more ascetic style of life embraced. There might be very good reasons why an individual might wish to embrace the ascetic, but they should preferably arise from an inner volition rather than being imposed by emotional blackmail.

For those unfortunate enough to suffer from a 'diet-related' disease, the implications of the thesis are even more forceful. How many victims of a heart attack wake up in the coronary-care unit of their local hospital to ponder the fact that a disease that will be with them for the rest of their lives has been caused by eating the wrong sort of food? No going back on that now. Heart disease is perceived as a self-induced illness and its victims have only themselves – or their mothers – to blame for putting eggs and bacon on the breakfast table three decades earlier. If and when they recover and it is time to leave hospital the dietary restrictions proposed by the diet-disease thesis have become imperative. Anxious to ward off a future heart attack, and taking courage from the belief that it is preventable if only the right magic formula of the diet is adopted, they willingly cut down on meat, substitute butter for a plastic bucket of polyunsaturated oils, and deny themselves salt on their vegetables. Anxiety compounds guilt; and to what purpose?

There are wider cultural implications of the diet-disease thesis than those of inducing neuroticism in the impressionable or the vulnerable, for it suggests there is something rotten at the core of Western civilisation. Forget that life expectancy is now greater than at any time in recorded history, that grinding poverty has all but been eliminated, that most now live better, freer, more interesting lives than at any other time. Understand instead that Western civilisation is corrupted and debilitated by its own affluence. Far from the virtues of our economic system being praised for having brought sufficiency to most, the very affluence is an indictment of that system, for it kills its citizens. The Marxist notion that capitalism is based on greed and acquisition acquires a specious validity from the annals of the diet-heart thesis, while fuelling whimsical fantasies of a better world.

The thesis might distort our image of the world but it also trivialises illness and death; it gives the public a totally misleading understanding of the nature of disease and evokes an inappropriate sense of doom. The reality that most live out their natural lifespan, only succumbing to complex diseases that medicine can alleviate but cannot cure, is transformed into the illusion that disease is ubiquitous, that its causes lie simply in the way we live and that they can be easily prevented. It fuels a fantasy that fate can be avoided and death postponed, and leads to completely inappropriate expectations of what medicine can achieve. While it is crucial for any profound moral intelligence to appreciate the seriousness of illness in human affairs, nothing is gained by becoming obsessed by human frailty. The diet-disease thesis, with its up-beat message of a long life through healthy eating, manages the double achievement of both trivialising the seriousness of illness, and making it appear too important by over-emphasising its role in life.

Perhaps the public is less impressed than all this would suggest. They have heard it all before. Doctors are so free with their advice on what is harmful in our lives that the sensible thing must be to carry on regardless. Scepticism and inertia become overwhelming virtues that keep the dismal admonitions of not very bright nutritional evangelists at bay. But what if the new nutritional wisdom is in itself actually harmful?

It is unlikely to be so. All the evidence shows that it matters little what people eat as long as they follow their appetites and instincts and are relatively sensible. If there remains a serious nutritional deficiency in some people's lives, it is a deficiency of money. So if under the onslaught of the thesis certain foods are rejected in favour of others, little harm will result.

There are, however, some theoretical dangers to consider. In an entirely sane world people would take the thesis more or less seriously and change their diet as they think appropriate. But the world is not entirely sane. There are some who find in food both a source of their unhappiness and the means with which to resolve that unhappiness. At its most extreme, this leads to food faddism which can result in serious nutritional deficiencies. The diet-disease thesis should not permit this sad folly, but perhaps the overt and highly publicised authoritarian emphasis on the importance of the role of food in illness might drive some towards the faddist camp who would not otherwise have travelled that path. This is particularly a danger when over-anxious parents, impressed by the 'harmfulness' of salt and dairy products, seek to guarantee the future health of their offspring by imposing on them restricted diets. There are reports of very young children whom low-salt diets have rendered relatively salt depleted and who become seriously ill when an acute episode of vomiting and diarrhoea critically reduces their body's store of this all-important mineral. The experts admit that the much-lauded low-fat/high-fibre diet is not suitable for very young children – for the obvious reason that it might restrict growth and predispose to rickets in the vulnerable – but are all those parents transfixed by the healthy diet message equally aware of this?

Again, perhaps the diet-disease thesis makes people inappropriately weary of all health education messages. It links in the public's mind certain foods with smoking and drinking as pleasurable activities that are to be actively discouraged. The very catholicity of these admonishments fail to discriminate those areas in which the evidence of benefit is powerful and convincing from those where it is not. It is conceivable that as a consequence some will fail to appreciate the imperative significance of quitting smoking for their future health. Overwhelmed by good advice, they do nothing and die from lung cancer.

In a similar vein, the thesis could distract from those activities which might have a useful impact in preventing heart disease, particularly exercise.[5] The mechanism of prevention is not entirely clear, although it is found in similar diseases. Just as those whose coronary arteries are narrowed by atheroma suffer from angina, so some get a condition known as 'peripheral vascular disease' in which the arteries to the legs are narrowed and limit the victim's ability to walk because not enough blood gets through to the leg muscles. If the patient takes regular but not excessive exercise the symptoms will often improve over a period of six months, probably because exercise opens up 'collateral' arteries through which more blood can flow to the previously blood-starved muscle. The same is likely to be true for heart disease. Those who take a lot of exercise have powerful heart muscles and adequate blood supply to those muscles. If whatever causes heart disease then strikes, the heart is better able to cope.

There are of course many good reasons for taking exercise, not the least being that it makes people feel better – so even if exercise does not prevent heart disease it would be of value. The point, however, is that by focusing on the lethality of food rather than the virtues of exercise the wrong public health message may be conveyed.

Furthermore, the emphasis on the dietary prevention of heart disease has almost certainly contributed to the severity of the epidemic in the Western world by distorting the whole emphasis of the research programme into the disease. Under the banyan tree nothing grows. Under the banyan tree of the diet-heart thesis no funds have been available for research into other possible causes. There is no guarantee that such research would have come up with an adequate explanation or indeed cure. But the epidemiology of the disease does strongly suggest there is a single unifying cause and nobody has bothered or perhaps been aware that it is worth looking for. The degree of ignorance about the disease is remarkable despite the enormous research effort into its causes. The source of this ignorance is not merely a lack of knowledge but arises from the complex forces that influence the pattern of research, as the late Professor Norman Geschwind of Harvard Medical School pointed out:

> There may be neglect of existing facts or theories, either through deliberate suppression or through widespread acceptance of incorrect data or erroneous criticisms. Furthermore though the actual lack of data in an important area should be a powerful stimulus to scientific curiosity, there are cases in which research is not carried out either because of the erroneous belief that there are no suitable investigative methods or because well-established scientists and administrators are unwilling to allocate resources to innovative areas because of timidity or simple desire to support their own fields at the expense of newer, less influential ones. Finally ignorance may result from the deliberate publication of false data, or the prevention of publication by rivals, or the wilful withholding of information that might enable others to move ahead.[6]

Finally, there is the damage done to the medical profession itself by the thesis. In the words of Professor J. R. A. Mitchell of Nottingham University:

> The harm which worries me is to our credibility as scientists and health advisers. . . . Over the centuries the public have been given so many crazy admonitions by 'leaders' of medical opinion (on the evils of masturbation, or constipation) that they cannot decide who to listen to and what they should do. If we fail in our duty to differentiate between what is known and has been proved and what is merely believed, then the harm from such false advice is to our credibility and to our self-esteem as scientists.[7]

But the harm goes deeper than the problem of credibility, to threaten the central heartspring of medical practice, the values of professional life. Medicine is, and has to be, a serious business. It deals with people at their most vulnerable and carries the dual responsibility of accurately diagnosing their illnesses and appropriately treating them. Error in either leads to further suffering and can be fatal. Doctors have to get it right. And they get it right by being guided not just by the vast corpus of knowledge that is 'medical science', but by having a discriminating scientific intellect based on a method that can distinguish illusion from reality and which is the only sure protection for the ill against the false solutions of quackery. Furthermore, when there is no cure or solution, a different type of intelligence is required, one that appreciates and can cope with the tragedies of people's lives.

These attributes are not universally found in society, but are to a greater or lesser extent found amongst doctors. They are not innate but are rather encouraged by membership of a self-regulating profession which promotes them by ensuring that ideas will be openly and freely discussed, that expertise is appreciated and excellence rewarded.

On several counts these professional virtues are threatened by the diet-disease thesis. Free and open discussion is not possible when important facts are withheld from the scientific argument – it is impossible to evaluate the validity of theories when their authority relies on the assertion of expert committees rather than the verdict of scientific experiment. The partisanship with which the diet-disease thesis has been promoted in the medical journals has set an unfortunate precedent where balanced argument has been replaced by a collection of facts selected merely to plead a case. Further, the thesis has convinced many doctors that much illness is self-induced, so that disease ceases to be a misfortune to which doctors must respond to the best of their ability and induces instead contempt for the way in which their patients lead their lives.

But most importantly, the thesis breaks down the self-regulating barriers of professional life by posing easy solutions that are taken up by many who are unaware of the subtleties and complexities of science. When the pronouncements of 'popular nutritionists' are given the same or greater weight as the sceptical observations of the best of the profession, the monkeys of ignorance run free over the exposed body of medicine and all values are corrupted.

References

1. Reasons for Doubt

1. Gordon T. 'Mortality experience among the Japanese in the United States, Hawaii & Japan', *Public Health Reports*, 1957, 72, 543–53.
2. Cornfield J. & Mitchell S. 'Selected risk factors in Coronary Disease', *Arch. Env. Hlth*, 1969, 19, 382–94.
3. *WHO Health Statistics Annual 1952–84*, WHO, Geneva.
4. *FAO Production Yearbook. 1982*, 36, FAO, Rome.
5. Codell Carter K. 'Koch's postulates in relation to the work of Jacob Henle and Edwin Klebs', *Medical History*, 1985, 29, 353–75.
6. Bradford Hill A. *A Short Textbook of Medical Statistics*, London, 1977.
7. Royal College of Physicians. *Smoking or Health*, London, 1977.

2. Fat is Harmful – Official

1. WHO. *Prevention of Coronary Heart Disease, WHO Technical Report Series*, No. 678, 1982, WHO, Geneva.
2. Bishop J. 'Heart Attacks: A Test Collapses', *Wall Street Journal*, 6 October 1982.
3. MRFIT Research Group. 'Multiple Risk Factor Intervention Trial', *JAMA*, 1982, 248, 1465–77.
4. WHO European Collaborative Group. 'Multifactorial Trial in the Prevention of Heart Disease, incidence and mortality results', *European Heart Journal*, 1983, 4, 141–7.
5. Editorial. 'Can I Avoid A Heart Attack?', *Lancet*, 1974, i, 605.
6. McMichael J. 'Dietetic Factors in Coronary Disease', *European Journal of Cardiology*, 1977, 5, 447–52.
7. Mann G. V. 'Diet–Heart, End of an Era', *NEJM*, 1977, 297, 644–50.

8. Ahrens E. H. 'Dietary Fats & Coronary Heart Disease, Unfinished Business', *Lancet*, 1979, ii, 1345–8.
9. NACNE. *Proposals for Nutritional Guidelines for Health Education in Britain*, HEC, London, 1983.
10. Health Education Council. *Coronary Heart Disease Prevention: Plans for Action*, London, 1984.
11. DHSS. *Diet & Cardiovascular Disease; Report on Health & Social Subjects No. 7*, HMSO, London, 1984.
12. British Medical Association. *Diet, Nutrition and Health*, BMA, London, 1986.
13. JACNE. *Eating for a Healthy Heart*, London, 1986.
14. European Atherosclerosis Society. 'Strategies for the Prevention of Coronary Heart Disease', *European Journal of Cardiology*, 1987, 8, 77–88.
15. Mitchell J. R. A. 'What constitutes evidence in the dietary prevention of Coronary Heart Disease? Cosy beliefs or harsh facts?', *International Journal of Cardiology*, 1984, 4, 287.
16. BBC. *Plague of Hearts*: BBC: *O'Donnell Investigates the Food Connection*; BBC: *Countdown to a Coronary*; Channel 4: *Food for Thought*.
17. Cannon G. & Walker C. *The Food Scandal*, London, 1984.
18. British Medical Association. *Nutrition and the Public Health*, BMA, London, 1939.

3. The Mysteries of Nutrition

1. McLaren D. S. *Nutrition & its Disorders*, London, 1981.
2. Owen O. E. *et al.* 'Ketone Body Metabolism in normal, obese & diabetic subjects', *Isr. J. Med.*, 1975, 11, 560–70.
3. Miller D. S., Mumford P. 'Gluttony', *Am. J. Clin. Nutr.*, 1967, 20, 1212–22.
4. Medical Research Council. *Special Report Series No. 274*, HMSO, 1951.
5. Durnin J. V. G. A. *et al.* 'How Much Food Does Man Require?', *Nature*, 1973, 212, 418.
6. Pacey A. & Payne P. (eds). *Agricultural Development & Nutrition*, London, 1985.
7. Watt J. 'Starving Sailors', 1981.
8. Magee H. E. 'Application of Nutrition to Public Health', *BMJ*, 30 March 1946, 475–81.
9. Cannon G. *The Times*, 12 June 1984.
10. Orr J. B. *Food, Health and Income*, London, 1936.
11. Corey Mann H. C. *Diets for Boys during School Age*. Medical Research Council, London, 1926.
12. Caroll K. K. 'Experimental Evidence of Dietary Factors

in Hormone Dependent Cancers', *Cancer Research*, 1975, 35, 3374–83.
13. Kelsey J. 'A Review of the Epidemiology of Human Breast Cancer', *Epidemiological Review*, 1979, 1, 74–109.

4. The Healthy Diet of 1936

1. Waugh E. *Vile Bodies*, London, 1936.
2. Orwell G. *Road to Wigan Pier*, London, 1937.
3. Hutt A. *The Condition of the Working Class in Britain*, London, 1933.
4. Loch Mowat C. *Britain Between the Wars 1918–40*, London, 1968.
5. 'A debate on Malnutrition', *Lancet*, 1936, ii, 156–8.
6. Orr J. B. *Food, Health and Income*, London, 1936.
7. McCarrison R. 'Nutrition & National Health', *BMJ*, 1936, 29 February, 427–30.
8. McCarrison R. 'Nutrition in Health and Disease', *BMJ*, 1936, 26 September, 611–15.
9. Codell Carter K. 'The Germ Theory, Beri Beri, and the Deficiency Theory of Disease', *Medical History*, 1977, 21, 119.
10. Castiglioni A. *A History of Medicine*, New York, 1847.
11. *Lancet*, 1930, ii, 1097.
12. Fletcher W. 'Rice and Beri Beri; preliminary report on an experiment conducted at the Kuala Lumpur Lunatic Asylum', *Lancet*, 1907, i, 1776–9.
13. Mellanby E. 'An experimental investigation on Rickets', *Lancet*, 1919, i, 202.
14. Paton R. 'Accessory Food Factors', *Proc. R. Soc. Med.*, 1920, 13, 77–86.
15. Medical Research Council. *Studies of Rickets in Vienna, 1919–22, MRC Special Report No.77*, 1923. HMSO, London.
16. Orr J. B., Gilks J. L. *Studies of Nutrition: The Physique & Health of Two African Tribes*, HMSO, London, 1931.
17. McCance R. A. & Widdowson E. M. *Breads White and Brown*, London, 1956.
18. Venner T. *Via Recta Ad Vitam Longam*, London, 1622.
19. Graham S. *A Treatise on Bread Making*, Boston, 1837.
20. Allinson T. R. *Medical Essays*, London, 1902.
21. Hutchinson R. *Food and the Principles of Dietetics*, London, 1906.
22. Editorial. *BMJ*, 1939, ii, 289.
23. Editorial. *Lancet*, 1941, i, 357.
24. 'Parliamentary Intelligence', *Lancet*, 1936, i, 747; 1936, ii, 1188; 1937, ii, 1109 and 1343.

25. Webster C. 'Healthy or Hungry Thirties', *History Workshop Journal*, 1982, No. 13, 110–29.

5. Words Without Knowledge

1. Magee H. E. 'Application of Nutrition to Public Health, Some Lessons of the War', *BMJ*, 1946, i, 1175–81.
2. Greaves J. P. & Hollingsworth D. F. 'Trends in Food Consumption in the UK', *World Rev. Nutr. Diet*, 1966, 6, 34–89.
3. Passmore R. & Robson J. S. (eds). *A Companion to Medical Studies*, chapter 44: 'Maternal & Perinatal Mortality & Morbidity'.
4. Medical Research Council. *Studies of Undernutrition in Wuppertal 1946–9, Special Report Series No. 275*, HMSO, London, 1951.
5. Widdowson E. M. & McCance R. A. *Studies on the nutritive value of bread and on the effect of variations in the extraction rate of flour on the growth of undernourished children, MRC Special Report Series No. 287*, HMSO, London, 1954.
6. McCance R. A. & Widdowson E. M. *Bread White and Brown*, London, 1956.
7. Carnegie United Kingdom Trust. *Family, Diet & Health in Prewar Britain*, Aberdeen, 1955.
8. McCance R. A. & Widdowson E. M. 'Food Tables, Their Scope and Limitations', *Lancet*, 1943, i, 230.
9. Wretkind A. 'Round table on comparison of dietary recommendations in different European countries', *Nutr. Metab.*, 1977, 21, 210–49.
10. *Annual Report of the Chief Medical Officer of the Ministry of Health*, 1932, 21–2; 1933, 208.
11. Hutchison R. 'The Nutrition Question', *Lancet*, 1936, i, 583–5.
12. Cathcart E. P. 'Food and Nutrition', *BMJ*, 1937, i, 583.
13. Batten L. W. 'Food and Health', *Lancet*, 1936, ii, 286.
14. Orr J. B. *Food and the People, Target for Tomorrow*, London, 1943.
15. The Royal Society. *Biographical Memoirs of Fellows of the Royal Society*, 1972, 18, 43–81.
16. McLaren D. S. 'A Fresh Look at Protein Calorie Malnutrition', *Lancet*, 1966, ii, 485–8.
17. McLaren D. S. 'The Great Protein Fiasco', *Lancet*, 1974, i, 93–6.
18. Brock J. F. *Monogram Series, WHO No. 8*, 1952.
19. Pyke M. *Myths about Nutrition, Symposium on Nutrition*, Royal College of Physicians of Edinburgh, 1980.
20. Waterlow J. C. & Payne P. R. 'The Protein Gap', *Nature*, 1979, 281, 250–1.

21. Stapleton D., Macdonald W. B. 'The Pathogenesis of Idiopathic Hypercalcaemia in Infancy', *Amer. J. Clin. Nutr.*, 1957, 5, 533.
22. British Paediatric Association Report, *BMJ*, 1964, i, 1659–61.

6. The Healthy Diet of 1980

1. Galbraith J. K. *The Affluent Society*, London, 1987.
2. Fries J. F. 'Ageing, Natural Death and the Compression of Morbidity', *NEJM*, 1980, 303, 130–5.
3. OPCS. *Annual Abstract of Statistics*, 1977.
4. OPCS. *Social Trends*. HMSO, London, 1983.
5. Open University. *T101, Living with Technology, Block 6, Health*, The Open University Press, 1971.
6. McKeown T. *The Role of Medicine*, Oxford, 1979.
7. *Dietary Goals for the United States*, US Govt. Printing Office, Washington, 1977.
8. National Advisory Council on Nutrition Education (NACNE). *Proposals for Nutritional Guidelines for Health Education*, London, 1983.
9. McMahon & Pugh. *Epidemiology*, Boston, Mass., 1970.
10. Stallones R. E. 'The Rise and Fall of Ischaemic Heart Disease', *Scientific American*, 1980, 243, 43–9.
11. Leibowitz J. O. *The History of Coronary Heart Disease*, Wellcome Institute of the History of Medicine, 1970.
12. McNee J. W. 'The Clinical Syndrome of Thrombosis of the Coronary Arteries', *QJM*, 1925, October, 44–51.
13. Cassidy M. 'Coronary Disease – The Harveian Oration', *Lancet*, 1946, ii, 587–90.
14. Brisson G. *Lipids in Human Nutrition*, MTP Press, 1982.
15. Ahrens E. H. *et al.* 'The Influence of Dietary Fats on Serum Lipids in Man', *Lancet*, 1957, i, 943–53.
16. Slack J. 'Risk of Ischaemic Heart Disease in Familial Hyperlipoproteinaemic States', *Lancet*, 1969, ii, 1380.
17. Brown M. S., Goldstein J. L. 'Familial Hypercholesteraemia, A Genetic Defect in the Low Density Lipoprotein Receptor', *NEJM*, 1976, 294, 1386–90.
18. Hilden T. *et al. Lancet*, 1961, ii, 327.
19. Medical Research Council. *BMJ*, 1964, 2, 837.
20. Mitchell J. R. A. *Advanced Medicine*, Vol. 17, chapter 20.

7. The Sources of Evidence

1. Kannel W. B. & Gordon T. *The Framingham Study. Some characteristics related to the incidence of cardiovascular disease and death. 18-Year Follow-up*, Publication 74–599. US Govt Printing Office, Washington, 1974.

2. Rose G. A. & Marmot M. G. 'Social Class and Coronary Heart Disease', *British Heart Journal*, 1981, 45, 13.
3. Keys A. *Seven Countries: a Multivariate Analysis of Death and Coronary Heart Disease*, Cambridge, Mass., 1980.
4. McGill H. C. Jr. *The Geographic Pathology of Atherosclerosis*, Baltimore, 1968.
5. Worth R. M. *et al.* 'Epidemiologic Studies of Coronary Heart Disease and Stroke in Japanese Living in Japan, Hawaii and California', *American Journal of Epidemiology*, 1975, 102, 481.
6. Lemon F. R., Walden R. T. 'Death from Respiratory System Disease among Seventh Day Adventist Men', *JAMA*, 1966, 198, 117.
7. Fraser G. *Preventive Cardiology*, Oxford, 1986, p. 7.
8. Doll R. & Peto R. *The Causes of Cancer*, Oxford, 1981.
9. Burkitt D. P., Trowell H. C. *Refined Carbohydrate Foods and Disease*, London, 1975.
10. Kellock B. *The Fibre Man*, London, 1985.
11. Hurt J. C. 'Sodium Intake and Hypertension, a Cause for Concern', *Annals of Internal Medicine*, May 1983, 724.

8. The Evidence Tested

1. MRFIT Research Group. 'Multiple Risk Factor Intervention Trial', *JAMA*, 1982, 248, 1465–77.
2. WHO European Collaborative Group. 'Multifactorial Trial in the Prevention of Heart Disease, Incidence and Mortality Results', *Eur. Heart. J.*, 1983, 4, 141–7.
3. Hjermann I. *et al.* 'Effect of Diet and Smoking Intervention on the Incidence of Coronary Heart Disease', *Lancet*, 1981, ii, 1303–10.
4. Lipid Research Clinic Programme. 'LRC–CPPT Results; Reduction in Incidence of Coronary Heart Disease', *JAMA*, 1984, 251, 351–6.
5. Salonen J. T., Puska P. *et al.* 'Decline in Coronary Heart Disease in Finland 1969–79', *BMJ*, 1983, 286, 1857–60.
6. Terris M. 'Epidemiology of Cirrhosis of the Liver – National Mortality data', *Am. J. Public Health*, 1967, 57, 2076–88.
7. *WHO Health Statistics Annual, 1952–84*, WHO, Geneva.
8. *FAO Production Yearbook, 1982*, FAO, Rome.
9. Friend G. *et al.* 'Food Consumption Patterns in the US, 1909–13 to 1976', in *Nutrition, Lipids and Coronary Heart Disease*, ed. R. Lawy, New York, 1979.
10. Stallones R. 'The Rise and Fall of Ischaemic Heart Disease', *Scientific American*, 1980, 243, 43–9.

9. Flaws in the Argument

1. Keys A. *Seven Countries: a Multivariate Analysis of Death and Coronary Heart Disease*, Cambridge, Mass., 1980.
2. Brisson G. *Lipids in Human Nutrition*, MTP Press, 1982, p. 98.
3. *WHO Health Statistics Annual, 1952–84*, WHO, Geneva.
4. Beese D. H. *Tobacco consumption in various countries. Tobacco Research Paper No. 6*, Tobacco Research Council, 1972.
5. US Public Health Services. *Health Consequences of Smoking. Public Health Service Publication No. 1696.*
6. Gordon T. 'Mortality Experience among the Japanese in the US, Hawaii and Japan', *Public Health Reports*, 1957, 72, 543–53.
7. Cornfeld J. & Mitchell S. 'Selected Risk Factors in Coronary Disease', *Arch. Env. Hlth*, 1969, 19, 382–94.
8. Locke & King. 'Cancer mortality amongst US Japanese', *JNCI*, 1980, 65, 1150–5.
9. Haenszel W. 'Cancer Mortality among the Foreign Born in the US', *JNCI*, 1961, 26, 37–127.
10. Marmot M. G. *et al.* 'Lessons from the Study of Immigrant Mortality', *Lancet*, 1984, i, 1455–7.
11. Tanaka H. *et al.* 'Secular Trends in Mortality from Cerebrovascular Disease in Japan, 1960–79', *Stroke*, 1982, 13, 61.
12. Garrawy W. M. *et al.* 'The Declining Incidence of Stroke', *NEJM*, 1979, 300, 449–52.
13. Hirayama T. 'Epidemiology of Cancer of the Stomach with specific reference to its recent decrease in Japan', *Cancer Research*, 1975, 35, 3460–3.
14. OPCS. *Trends in Mortality, 1951–75 in England and Wales*, Series DH1 No. 3, HMSO, London.
15. Lewis B. *Environment, Metabolic Systems and Public Health. Oxford Textbook of Public Health*, Oxford, 1985.
16. Lemon F. R., Walden R. T. 'Death from Respiratory System Disease among Seventh Day Adventist Men', *JAMA*, 1966, 198, 117.
17. Lyon J. L. 'Cardiovascular Mortality in Mormons and Non-Mormons in Utah 1969–71', *Am. J. Epid.*, 1978, 108, 357–65.
18. Barker D. & Osmond C. 'Diet and Coronary Heart Disease in England and Wales during and after the Second World War', *J. Epid. & Comm. Hlth*, 1986, 4037–44.
19. Strom A. 'Mortality from Circulatory Disease in Norway 1940–5', *Lancet*, 1951, i, 126–9.
20. Morris J. N. 'Recent History of Coronary Disease', *Lancet*, 1951, i, 69–73.
21. Crawford T. & Crawford M. 'Prevalence and Pathological Changes of Ischaemic Heart Disease in a Hard Water and in a Soft Water Area', *Lancet*, 1967, i, 229–32.

22. Lillienfield A. M. 'The Humean Fog; Cancer and Cholesterol', *Am. J. Epid.*, 1981, 114, 1–10.
23. Rose G. 'Plasma Lipids and Mortality, a Source of Error', *Lancet*, 1980, i, 523–6.
24. Cummings J. H. 'Health and the Large Intestine', *Nutrition and Health*, ed. M. Turner, MTP Press, 1982.

10. A Serious Deception

1. MRFIT Research Group. 'Multiple Risk Factor Intervention Trial', *JAMA*, 1982, 248, 1465–77.
2. Stallones R. E. 'Mortality and the MRFIT Trial', *Am. J. Epid.*, 1983, 117, 647–50.
3. WHO European Collaborative Group. 'Multifactorial Trial in the Prevention of Coronary Heart Disease', *Eur. Ht. J.*, 1983, 4, 141–7.
4. Lipid Research Clinic Programme. 'LRC-CPPT Results', *JAMA*, 1984, 251, 351–6.
5. Cholesterol study in US hailed as 'landmark', *International Herald Tribune*, 19 January 1984.
6. 'Giving Cholesterol a Bad Name', *Newsweek*, 23 January, 1984.
7. Rose G. 'Strategy of Prevention; Lessons from Cardiovascular Disease', *BMJ*, 1981, 282, 1847–51.
8. Oliver M. 'Should we not forget about mass control of coronary risk factors?' *Lancet*, 1983, ii, 37.
9. 'Lowering Blood Cholesterol to Prevent Heart Disease', *JAMA*, 1985, 253, 2080–93.
10. Oliver M. 'Consensus or Nonsensus conference on Coronary Heart Disease', *Lancet*, 1985, i, 1087.
11. Ahrens E. H. 'The Diet-Heart question in 1985; has it really been settled?' *Lancet*, 1985, i, 1085.
12. Marmot M. G. *et al.* 'Changes in Heart Disease Mortality in England and Wales and other countries', *Health Trends*, 1981, 13.
13. Rose G. *Cardiovascular Disease, Oxford Textbook of Public Health*, Oxford, 1985.
14. NACNE. *Proposals for Nutritional Guidelines for Health Education in Britain*, HEC, London, 1983.
15. Swales J. *Salt and High Blood Pressure; A Study in Education Persuasion and Naivety. A Diet of Reason*. Social Affairs Unit, 1986.
16. Brown J. J. & Lever *et al. Lancet*, 1984, ii, 456.
17. Svanborg A. *et al.* 'Comparison of Ecology, Ageing and State of Health in Japan and Sweden', *Acta Med. Scand.*, 1985, 218, 5–17.

12. Final Meditations

1. Mencius. *Mencius*, tr. D. C. Lau, London, 1970.
2. Djilas M. *Conversations with Stalin*, London, 1962.
3. Athanaeus. *The Deipnosophists*, tr. C. D. Yonge, London, 1854.
4. Goody J. *Cooking, Cuisine and Class, a Study in Comparative Sociology*, Cambridge, 1982.
5. Morris J. N. 'Vigorous exercise in leisure time and the incidence of Coronary Heart Disease', *Lancet*, 1973, i, 333–9.
6. Geschwind N. 'The neglect of advances in the Neurology of Behaviour', *The Encyclopaedia of Medical Ignorance*, ed. R. Duncan & M. Weston Smith, London, 1984.
7. Mitchell J. R. A. 'What constitutes evidence in the dietary prevention of Coronary Heart Disease – Cosy beliefs or harsh facts?' *Int. J. Cardiol.*, 1984, 4, 287.

Index

Uganda, 95
Unilever, 144–6
United States of America, 80, 91;
    decline in heart disease, 6–10,
    106–7, 110–11, 113, 138, 155;
    fat consumption, 110–11;
    migrant studies, 4–6, 10, 96,
    122–3; Prohibition, 107;
    Seventh Day Adventists, 93–4,
    116, 125–6, 127
US Congress, 80
US National Institute of Health,
    136–7

varicose veins, 130
vegetarians, 93–4, 116, 125–6,
    127
Vienna, 48–9, 59
viruses, 151
vitamins, 66, 69; deficiencies, 3,
    10, 31–2, 45–50, 154;
    supplements, 73–5
vitamin A, 32, 63, 64, 96

vitamin B group, 65
vitamin B (thiamin), 45, 47, 51,
    56, 73
vitamin C, 31, 32, 42, 57
vitamin D, 32, 45, 47, 49, 54, 57,
    74–5, 156

Walker, Caroline, 22
Wall Street Journal, 16
warfarin, 88
Widdowson, Elsie, 59–61
Winkler, 46
womb cancer, 96, 130
World Food Board, 70, 73
World Health Organization
    (WHO), 16–18, 23, 103, 105,
    133, 134, 135, 136, 138
Wuppertal, 59–61

xerophthalmia, 32

Yugoslavia, 91–2, 110, 118